How Brain Arousal Mechanisms Work

How Brain Arousal Mechanisms Work

Paths Toward Consciousness

Donald Pfaff
The Rockefeller University

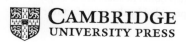

CAMBRIDGE
UNIVERSITY PRESS

CAMBRIDGE
UNIVERSITY PRESS

University Printing House, Cambridge CB2 8BS, United Kingdom

One Liberty Plaza, 20th Floor, New York, NY 10006, USA

477 Williamstown Road, Port Melbourne, VIC 3207, Australia

314–321, 3rd Floor, Plot 3, Splendor Forum, Jasola District Centre, New Delhi – 110025, India

79 Anson Road, #06-04/06, Singapore 079906

Cambridge University Press is part of the University of Cambridge.

It furthers the University's mission by disseminating knowledge in the pursuit of education, learning, and research at the highest international levels of excellence.

www.cambridge.org
Information on this title: www.cambridge.org/9781108433334
DOI: 10.1017/9781108377485

First published 2019

Printed and bound in Great Britain by Clays Ltd, Elcograf S.p.A.

A catalogue record for this publication is available from the British Library.

ISBN 978-1-108-43333-4 Paperback

Dedicated to the work and memory of Professor Fred Plum, M.D.

Contents

Acknowledgments

Insofar as this book puts forth a clear and well-reasoned set of arguments, the help of lawyer and former English professor Sandra Sherman must be recognized.

Thanks to Anna Whiting at the Cambridge University Press for conceiving of neuroscience books which contribute to neurology and to Nigel Graves, of the Press, for managing its production with great efficiency.

All of the book has benefited from the critical readings and suggestions from professors, to whom I am as grateful as a person can be. Professors Larry Abbott (Columbia), Jayanth Banavar (Oregon) and Randy Gallistel (Rutgers), Chapters 1, 10, and the Introduction; Peggy Mason (Chicago), Chapter 2; Clif Saper (Harvard), Chapters 3 and 4; Jack Feldman (University of California, Los Angeles), Chapter 3; James Herman (Cincinnati), Chapter 4; Rae Silver (Columbia), H. L. Haas (Heinrich-Heine University Düsseldorf, Duesseldorf, Germany) and Laszlo Zaborszky (Rutgers), Chapter 5; David Amaral (University of California Davis) and Avi Snyder (Washington University, St. Louis), Chapter 6; Randy Nelson (Ohio State) and Michael Baum (Boston University), Chapter 7; and Alex Proekt (Pennsylvania) and Peter Forgacs (Cornell), Chapter 8.

To all of these experts I am more than thankful.

Introduction

This is a book written with a depth of literature review that should appeal to neurologists interested in the application of basic science to their profession. In addition, the text tries for a clarity that should invite a look by educated non-scientists.

To reverse engineer brain arousal mechanisms, I reframe a vital question with a formulation not previously used: "*Why does any animal or human do anything at all*"?

Beyond citing facts, I propose theoretical ideas about how brain arousal systems are organized. They must be reliable and they are. First, the nerve cell groups which support arousal are highly interconnected. In particular, some "master neurons" for arousal have such long axons sporting additional projections short, medium, and long that the neural net for what I call Generalized Arousal (GA) looks to me scale-free; that is, lots of neurons have few connections but these "master cells" have an extremely large number of connections. And the GA system can produce scale-free behavior. Thinking this way offers the opportunity of applying the rigor of physical and mathematical approaches to neurological and behavioral science. Because these master cells are supplying identical signals over their long axons up and down the neuraxis, they are, necessarily, producing "neuronal integration." Because these long axons run up (anterior) and down (posterior) the neuraxis, we therefore can talk about an anterior/posterior longitudinal integrated (A/P,L integrated) arousal system. As this system evolved from fishes to humans, it developed a high road (through the thalamus) as well as a low road (through the hypothalamus) from the brainstem to the forebrain. Both are important.

Chapters will follow this A/P, L integrated system from the hindmost brainstem cell groups – embryologically the myencephalon (medulla) – through the metencephalon (pons) and mesencephalon (midbrain) to see how arousing signals are sent through the "low road" (hypothalamus) and the "high road" (thalamus) to activate the forebrain.

This book is *not* a philosophical contemplation upon consciousness. It pits forth a theory which explains how all of us manage a phase transition from deep anesthesia, from deep sleep, or from traumatic brain injury into the dawn, the first light of consciousness.

Biological theorists who seek to explain consciousness have gotten stuck in the cerebral cortex, citing it as the *situs* of consciousness, i.e., where consciousness arises. I will challenge this notion and, accordingly, offer a new theory of how we become conscious during various natural or induced states in which we are unconscious. My approach will not limit activity bearing on consciousness to the cortex – or to any single element of the central nervous system (CNS) – but, rather, will take into account operations in an

Dedicated to the memory of the distinguished neurologist Fred Plum.

array of neuronal structures. My purpose is to provide a better physical understanding of paths toward consciousness, and thereby enhance the ability of medical and neuroscience personnel to treat individuals whose physical consciousness is the desired goal.

Two leading theorists exemplify what I would call the cortico-centric tendency in the study of consciousness. The first, Giulio Tononi, a renowned neuroscientist in the Department of Psychiatry at the University of Wisconsin School of Medicine, has presented what he terms the "integrated information theory" of consciousness. The theory seems to offer unnecessary formalisms to explain the obvious, while failing to explain the causative routes of consciousness in the CNS. For example, he states that "a physical system in a state with high (integrated information) necessarily has many elements and specifies many causal relationships" (Marshall et al., 2016). The theory does not really provide mechanisms – it just pushes back the problem one step. When he experiments by tracking "changes in resting-state functional connectivity between wake and slow wave sleep," he does not need this theory at all (Deco et al., 2014). This "integrated" information theory does not provide a mechanism. It simply pushes the problem back one step – what kind of information? what exactly is integration? Professor Tononi simply names the goal; he does not get there.

In some of Tononi's theoretical work, he collaborates with a prominent researcher on the visual cortex, Christof Koch. When Koch was a professor at Caltech, he was stimulated to work on "the hard problem," consciousness, by the charismatic Nobel laureate Sir Francis Crick. While Koch and Tononi recognize that ever longer lists of "correlations between the behavioural and neuronal features of experience" (Tononi and Koch, 2015) will not suffice to explain causative routes to consciousness, they still feel the need to resort to "integrated information theory" with respect to cortical function and consciousness. This seems to beg the question, since it does not broach how the CNS, as a system, produces consciousness.

In the context of explaining consciousness, the term "integrated information theory" presents a problem of transparency. In that theory, only "information" can be defined precisely in mathematical terms, as in Claude Shannon's well-known 1948 information equation (see Chapter 10). Tononi's approach amounts to a top-down theory. In a top-down theory the scientist deduces properties of a system from first, abstract principles, i.e., from an overview. Once in a while top-down works. For example, in 1943, MIT's Warren McCulloch and Walter Pitts proved what could be deduced about neural nets using only "the two-valued logic of propositions" (p. 133). But usually neuroscientists theorize from the bottom-up. A bottom-up system starts with experimental details and induces how they can be pieced together to form subsystems and (larger, more inclusive) systems.

Here I use the bottom-up approach, literally bottom up, starting in the lower brainstem (Pfaff et al., 2005, 2008), where large reticular neurons provide the essential driving force for elevated levels of CNS arousal. For this approach, we arrive at the cerebral cortex only after the operations of extended A/P signaling through several modules which will be explained in this book. Thus we strive to reframe thinking about CNS arousal and consciousness by conceiving *a long anterior/posterior longitudinal ladder-like (A/P,L) system that is vertically integrated,* by virtue of a scale-free network, with each module in the system coding for a different essential physiological property of the system. The long A/P connections serve to combine separate elements, to form a complete, coordinated entity – i.e., to achieve an integrated GA system.

In this regard, the Nobel prize-winning physicist Richard Feynman once said that he could not really understand a physical phenomenon unless he could put it together himself, that is, reconstruct it from basic elements. An intellectually gratifying feature of studying CNS arousal systems is that we can, indeed, reconstruct, i.e., faithfully duplicate, the elementary steps of increased arousal by electrical and chemical manipulations of arousal pathways.

We not only know where those pathways are, we also know what they do.

Instead of being limited to individual neuronal regions, "centers" for CNS arousal, I focus on long, A/P systems of communication that support the initiation of behavioral acts and, indeed, consciousness. Such systems do not originate in the cerebral cortex. Electrical and metabolic activity in the cortex represent the ultimate expression of successful function of neuronal signaling systems that begin just above the spinal cord. Every bit of arousal and awareness, every thought, has an underlying cause resident in the function of these extended neuronal systems.

This book will offer a new view of how these systems work. Strung along the long A/P pathways are large modules, neuronal groups that process arousal-related signaling and add unique functions and features. These will be explained, chapter by chapter.

Consciousness. As I mentioned, the deepest roots of consciousness (e.g., the first onset of awareness as the brain moves from the null states of coma, deep anesthesia, or deep sleep) lie far posterior in the hindbrain, not just in the cerebral cortex where most people think they lie. In the hindbrain reticular formation, certain large neurons essential for initiating brain arousal and consciousness are found just above the spinal cord. These large neurons had their evolutionary origins in the fish brain and have their developmental origins on the surfaces of the embryonic brain.

Of course, as a neuroscientist I take a reductionist approach to the term "conscious," and address the *physical* elements of consciousness precedent to the fullest intellectual interpretations of the subject. For example, this book does not deal with states of deep contemplation, nor does it deal with philosophical speculations on the relationship between self and world.

Instead, I emphasize that neuroscientists are studying the most fundamental, elemental, primitive entries into consciousness. The writing here presents the physical realization of mechanisms which lay out in neurobiological and molecular detail how arousal pathways work, how they "wake up the brain" as from deep anesthesia, coma, or sleep.

Modules. The chapter order is linear, moving from hindbrain to forebrain and then from animal brain to human brain. Each chapter will take up an element of that idea, always building on the preceding chapter to produce a unified approach to our new understanding of brain arousal mechanisms necessary for consciousness.

Chapters

1. **Concept.** Some years ago, in *Brain Arousal and Information Theory,* I proposed the concept of Generalized CNS (central nervous system) Arousal (GA). The book presented an operational definition of GA and listed GA's operating requirements. Physicist Jayanth Banaver and I theorized that the passage from low GA to high GA had characteristics of a physical phase transition. Quantitative assays for measuring GA are available for experimental animals and patients. Many years of new data on arousal mechanisms have led us to focus on large reticular formation nerve cells,

"Nucleus Giganto Cellularis" (NGC) as the most powerful and essential neurons for initiating GA.

2. **NGC.** Experimentally elevating activity in these large reticular formation neurons activates the electrical activity of the cerebral cortex and initiates movements, even in deeply anesthetized animals. My lab have just discovered the entire transcriptome of one subclass of these neurons, among the "master cells" of CNS arousal, neurons whose axons project to the central thalamus (see Chapter 6). NGC neurons express genes for receptors of neurotransmitters and neuropeptides known to modulate GA.

   Since these neurons represent the origins of arousal, the physical location where arousal originates, I can, in this chapter, put forward the "origins of the origins of arousal" (i) in evolutionary terms, and (ii) during early brain development; and (iii) first awakenings just after birth.

   The next four chapters move up the neuraxis toward the forebrain, and will describe the physiology and genetic studies available at each of the four levels.

3. **Pons.** Just in front of NGC neurons are large neurons in the pons that regulate sleep. Their chemistry has been elucidated and their electrophysiology well described. Working on two nearby cell groups, Karolinska Institutet professor Ole Kiehn has discovered how chemically defined neurons at the anterior border of the pons regulate the initiation of locomotor behaviors.

4. **Midbrain.** Harvard professor Clifford Saper has laid out the neuroanatomy and physiology of opposing nerve cell groups in the pons and midbrain, one of which elevates arousal while the other decreases arousal.

   Pathways ascending from the midbrain will split into a "low road" and a "high road." The low road addresses the large cholinergic neurons of the basal forebrain. Those are the neurons that are helped by Alzheimers-delaying medications. The high road addresses the central thalamus, where electrical stimulation has caused a patient with a disorder of consciousness to regain consciousness.

5. **Hypothalamus.** Hypothalamic neurons receive signals from the low road. They include neuroendocrine neurons that regulate hormones associated with GA. Importantly, they also include the huge cholinergic neurons of the basal forebrain.

   A unique group of GA neurons express the gene for hypocretin/orexin (same gene, cloned and named by two labs). The gene product fosters higher GA especially when connected with hunger. Mutations in this gene or either of its two receptors leads to narcolepsy, a sudden and temporary loss of posture and consciousness.

6. **Central Thalamus.** These neurons receive signals from the high road. They participate with essential roles in a specific forebrain circuit named a "mesocircuit" by neurology professor Nicholas Schiff. High levels of activity in this circuit are required for purposeful movement. Electrical stimulation of central thalamic neurons by Schiff caused a high-end vegetative patient to regain consciousness.

7. **High arousal states.** This chapter will summarize succinctly what is known about mechanisms for sex behaviors, fear, and aggression and show how they are linked to and depend on GA.

8. **Low arousal states.** The chapter explores the medical analyses of coma, deep anesthesia, and deep sleep. Emergence from these "zero states" requires elevation of GA.

9. **Aroused, conscious.** Neurophysiological and molecular biological supports for GA obviously feed into mechanisms underlying consciousness in the human brain. But how much farther can we go from a neuroscientific understanding of GA toward the elements of consciousness? As a skeptical scientist, I will argue that some philosophical approaches to the so-called "mind–brain problem" smack of the paradoxes of self-reference illustrated by Bertrand Russell (e.g., "This sentence is wrong").

10. **A vertically integrated system.** Obviously, some of the outstanding properties of GA systems are linked to each other. The length of axons in an A/P,L system with synaptic connections at several levels allows a high degree of connectivity and, because of these large neurons, raises the possibility of a scale-free system. The large NGC neurons – with widespread dendrites, lengthy projections, multimodal sensitivity, and high firing rates – exemplify neurons with incredibly large channel capacity, sending an integrated signal up and down the neuraxis.

Visions for where work on GA in animal brains will go tend to concentrate on how new genetic and epigenetic knowledge will be integrated with the neural circuitry understanding which we already have. Regarding neurologists' work with human consciousness, I will concentrate on high-end vegetative states because patients in those states require the most attention and represent the greatest opportunities.

There emerges the picture of a bilaterally symmetric A/P,L integrated long-axon scale-free system in which its high degree of connectivity enforces its physiological power.

For the first time, neuroscientists are closing in on a comprehensive understanding of brain arousal pathways and mechanisms that are essential for consciousness. Hopefully these neuroscientific efforts will augment the progress already made on the crushingly severe problems of disorders of consciousness by pioneering neurologists (Laureys and Schiff, 2012; Laureys, 2016a,b; Bodart et al., 2017; Chennu et al., 2017). This book considers the physical manifestation of how traditional neuroanatomical results with regard to this topic are now complemented by neurophysiological and molecular genetic work. From those large reticular neurons mentioned above, a "low road" ascends deeper in the brain, through the hypothalamus and a "high road" through the thalamus ascends to the forebrain to support brain arousal. All of these basic neuroscience results support a new understanding of the deepest elements of human consciousness.

Here, then, the idea is to take a hard problem, consciousness, and in the interest of precisely determining brain mechanisms, to restate and reduce part of that problem to a smaller piece, that is, to ask "how do animals and human beings initiate behavior?" What are the physical paths toward consciousness? The general principles that I propose in response to that question will likely hold true universally for all vertebrates.

Chapter 1

Concept

Why does a human or any vertebrate animal do anything at all? In the central nervous system (CNS), what accounts for the initiation of behavior – any behavior, from the simplest to the most complex? And how universal an answer to these questions can we achieve?

Of course, some behavioral responses are reflexes triggered automatically by compelling stimuli – for example, in response to touching fire a person will quickly withdraw his hand. This book does not concern reflexes, or similar automatic actions that are not indicia of emerging consciousness.

Among non-reflexive behavior patterns, virtually all are motivated, directly or indirectly, by some state of body or mind. In many cases, these are obvious: hunger, thirst, fear, sex, anger. Equally obvious are states of mind such as motivations to achieve, compete, look good, or help others. If we think of these as "forces," neuronal modulations that increase the probabilities of certain kinds of behavioral patterns, then it is easy to understand that entire fields of neuroscience are devoted to how these motivational systems work – specific forces, specific behaviors.

But now we get to the issue that drives this book. Does there exist, at a level deeper than these specific motivational forces and prior to them in the causal chains for behavior, a powerful nonspecific influence? Yes. It is a concept, an influence that I have named "generalized CNS arousal" (GA) (Pfaff, 2006). Theoretically, GA would be very important to understand and regulate because it would contribute to the excitation of a wide range of behaviors. Correspondingly, its dysregulation would cause tremendous cognitive and emotional dysfunction.

Suppose, as argued below, GA does indeed exist. In this context, and inspired by the considerations outlined above, I want to reframe our thinking, and conceive a vertically integrated, ladder-like anterior/posterior longitudinal (A/P, L) network that produces GA. The integration likely comes about from a scale-free network – many neurons with small numbers of connections, as well as a few neurons, including those highlighted in these chapters, with very large numbers of connections.

I am thinking about GA differently from what has for a long time been the conventional approach to arousal, i.e., its *situs* is in the cortex. However, while GA is exciting to contemplate, it was also initially scary to conjecture, since up until not too long ago my scientific efforts were devoted to understanding very specific, simple behaviors such as sex and maternal behaviors (Pfaff, 2017). The most encouraging thing that happened along the way to my initial conjecture was that I could cross the street to learn about consciousness from a world authority on the disorders of consciousness, Professor Fred

Plum, Chief of Neurology at Cornell Medical School. This book is dedicated to Dr. Plum. But even so, understanding of arousal systems at that time was still couched in pure neurology and pure neurophysiology. That is, neurologists would consider the effects of certain kinds of damage – strokes, cardiac events, traumatic brain injuries – on the cognitive capacities of patients. Neurophysiologists knew that certain kinds of electrical stimuli in the brainstem could cause the appearance of higher frequencies of electrical wave activity recorded at the cerebral cortex and that major brainstem damage would have the opposite effect (Dempsey and Morison, 1942a, b; Lindsley et al., 1949; Moruzzi and Magoun, 1949; Magoun book, 1958). But I wanted to think differently about brain arousal mechanisms.

In order to "think differently," one can ask whether it is possible to construct a set of ideas about CNS arousal that would have a degree of precision and generality – even universality – that is more typical of physical than biological science. That is, physicists have been able to refer to physical principles that hold true under wide varieties of circumstances, and they could say to biologists "you guys don't have principles, but only Latin names and long lists of phenomena to memorize." In this vein, this book offers a precise and universal *operating definition* of CNS arousal, discussed as follows:

Operational definition: A more aroused animal or human, with higher GA, is more alert to sensory stimuli in many sensory modalities (S), more active motorically (M), and more reactive emotionally (E).

What about *operating requirements*? To start, at least four requirements can be justified on a theoretical basis: (i) GA mechanisms must work fast enough to allow the individual to escape danger, (ii) there must be great convergence of inputs onto GA mechanisms so that a wide variety of incoming signals can trigger adequate behavioral responses, (iii) there must be great divergence of signals emanating from GA mechanisms so that a wide variety of behavioral responses can be initiated, and (iv) GA mechanisms must be robust enough so that they will not fail (Pfaff et al., 2012).

As conceived, GA mechanisms work in all vertebrate brains including, of course, the human brain.

Within this definition and set of operating requirements, GA is fundamental to all cognitive functions. For example, you can be aroused without being alert, but not alert without being aroused. You can be alert without paying attention, but not the reverse. This holds true on up the chain of more complex cognitive states, all dependent on GA.

Likewise, GA is essential for all emotional expression. Whether a person is exhibiting a certain range of emotions momentarily (feelings), over hours (moods), or over a lifetime (temperament), the nature of the emotion depends on the situation, but the *strength* of expression depends on GA. If you think of emotional expression as a vector, the angle of the vector depends on the exact feeling but the length of the vector is determined, in part, by the level of GA.

Of course, since GA is so basic to cognitive and emotional functions, when something goes wrong with its mechanisms the organism can be thrown into chaos. Some of the maladies that can result are discussed below.

Other properties of CNS arousal systems have become evident over decades of research (Pfaff, 2006). Five of them are discussed in the following:

Bilaterality. In contrast to sensory and motor systems, for which directionalities of stimuli and responses are, essentially, the "name of the game," there is no need for sidedness in CNS arousal. In fact, it would be hard to imagine a life in which one half of a brain is more capable of arousal than the other.

Unilateral damage to the brain is unlikely to cause coma. Unilateral damage can cause asymmetry in the electrical activity of the cerebral cortex, as displayed in the electro-encephalogram (EEG), but it does not cause coma (Kushida ref 660 in 2006).

In the words of Steven Laureys (2016a, b), absence of arousal and awareness results from "diffuse bihemispheric cortical damage or from focal but extensive brain stem lesions" (3346). See also the work of Bartolomeo and Chokron (2002), a neurologist at INSERM Unit 324 in Paris, dealing with patients who are conscious but who have received unilateral damage to their posterior cerebral cortex. If the damage was on the right side of the cerebral cortex, they would tend to ignore objects on their left, objects that would otherwise be seen. However, the situation is not entirely symmetric. If the damage was on the left side, attentional processes "seem to be relatively preserved, if slowed, in left unilateral neglect." The reason for the difference is not known. In any case, the idea of a bilateral arousal system is clearly accurate.

There are many unanswered questions about how the two sides of an arousal system work together. The next chapter focuses on what can be called the "master cells" for arousal deep in the hindbrain reticular formation. What will happen if we do new experiments in which only the left or only the right side of these cell populations are selectively stimulated or inhibited by specially designed viral vectors? Will behavioral responses be one-sided, or will they be bilaterally symmetrical? New studies of gait control by Veronique VanderHorst at Harvard Medical School, presented at the annual meeting of the Society for Neuroscience, suggest specific one-sided and nuanced contributions by medullary reticular neurons, but many neuroanatomical studies predict bilateral symmetry. By the way, up and down the long anterior/posterior longitudinal (A/P, L) systems emphasized in the book, many neurons project from the left side of the brainstem to the right, and *vice versa*. A first guess regarding their function is that they add stability to arousal systems. Particularly, if one side is damaged, signals from the other could compensate. But that is not known. These are open questions.

Anterior/posterior longitudinal (A/P, L) bidirectionality. Long A/P, L, ladder-like signaling forms the backbone of CNS arousal signaling. Its features are easiest to think about in that they comprise activation of neurons in more posterior ("lower") neuronal groups projecting ("ascending") to more anterior ("higher") neuronal groups. Consequently, signals will reach the hypothalamus, the thalamus, and the cerebral cortex. This is the textbook view of arousal systems neurophysiology (Kandel, 2000; Squire et al., 2008).

Arousal levels depend on the state of excitation of this long A/P, L network. Just think of one example: the long and widely distributed axons ascending from a noradrenergic cell group, locus coeruleus, in the pons, comprises cells that release noradrenalin (also known as norepinephrine) in the forebrain (e.g., Aston-Jones et al., 2001).

The reverse scenario is equally interesting. Clif Saper, now professor of neurology at Harvard Medical School, demonstrated axonal projections from the anterior hypothalamus all the way to the spinal cord (Saper et al., 1976). In my lab, graduate student Lily Conrad used radioactively labeled amino acids microinjected into the hypothalamus or into neuronal groups just in front of the hypothalamus to make radioactive proteins that could be followed as they traveled down axons descending to the lower brainstem (Conrad and Pfaff, 1975; Conrad et al., 1976a, b). Most startling, scientists in Arthur Loewy's lab at Washington University in Saint Louis used special viruses that are transported across synapses to demonstrate connections from preoptic neurons in the basal forebrain all the way to sympathetic autonomic ganglia in the abdomen.

The great Spanish neuroanatomist Valverde (1961) used the silver stain, discovered by Camillo Golgi, and exploited brilliantly by Ramon and Cajal, to study the morphology and explore the logic of long A/P, L systems of the brainstem (see Figure 2.2). While his (and my) most intense focus is on the human brain, his basic conclusions would hold true for all mammals. Valverde charted both long axonal systems that run up and down the A/P, L axis of the brainstem and short connections, i.e., short collaterals at right angles to the long axons. He pictures the operation of a "multiple chain system" (Valverde, 1961, 1962), by which he means that parallel A/P, L running axons start at different points in the neuraxis, end at different points, and probably overlap in their functions but are not identical. In this system, specificity of signaling would seem impossible.

Another leading group that used the Golgi stain concurs (Scheibel and Scheibel, 1961; Hobson and Scheibel, 1980; Jasper, 1958). They also emphasized long A/P, L connectivity in what they called "the reticular core" of the brainstem, coupled with extensive collateral protrusions perpendicular to the A/P, L axis where there would be contact with local dendrites. My neuroanatomy professor at MIT, Walle J. H. Nauta, taught us that the phylogenetically primitive reticular core extended from the intermediate nerve cell groups of the posterior spinal cord, through the upper spinal cord, through the lower brainstem, forward to the hypothalamus and central thalamus. Connections with local nerve cells would be intense because the very broad dendritic spreads are shaped in a so-called "isodendritic" tree (Ramon-Moliner and Nauta, 1966). In such a tree, the first dendritic segment sticking out from the nerve cell body would be shorter than the second, which is shorter in turn than the third segment (opposite to the so-called "allodendritic" tree, typical specific sensory relay pathways).

This situation can give rise to the network structure highlighted by physicist Albert-Laszlo Barabási (2002, 2009). In this type of network, large numbers of neurons have small numbers of connections, close by, whereas just a few neurons have large numbers of connections, in our case with arousal systems, distributed along the A/P, L axis of the brainstem. Chapter 2 discusses these latter neurons, with large numbers of A/P, L connections.

Still another property of the primitive reticular core has just been discovered by Inna Tabansky in my lab at Rockefeller (Tabansky et al., 2018). As discussed in Chapter 2, she listed the genes expressed by certain large reticular neurons in the posterior hindbrain, i.e., the medulla just above the spinal cord, and found a gene with a product that can operate on blood vessels. Further, these same neurons are right next to blood vessels with no intervening cells. A small amount of preliminary evidence also suggests that some of these medullary reticular neurons can sense chemicals in the blood; thus, they may be called "chemosensors." Exactly what this discovery means for the regulation of CNS arousal remains to be worked out.

Response potentiation. Most of the time, higher generalized arousal prepares the animals or human beings to initiate a behavioral response to stimuli of all sensory modalities, initiate voluntary locomotion, and react with feeling to emotional challenges. The trickiest interpretation of this idea is when a vertebrate is responding to a stimulus that indicates danger and "freezes." Under such circumstances, when for example a person is walking along, relaxed, and then freezes because of a danger ahead, the ostensible nonreaction would be considered an active behavioral response.

Sensitivity combined with stability. It is clear that changes in CNS arousal systems must, under some circumstances, cause the brain and body to rapidly achieve change of states. Yet they must also function within defined limits, and have the capacity to return to base-line. These two properties would seem to oppose each other, and we do not know yet how the balance between them is achieved. What are the critical arousal network features that shape the performance of the CNS through time? To address this question, we (Bubnys et al., in press) are trying to simulate such systems to ask the "what-if" questions imagina-tively and rapidly.

Some aspects of arousal system stability may derive from opposing actions both at the electrophysiological level and at the transcriptional level. As to the former, in parts of the A/P, L extended CNS arousal system, excitatory glutamatergic neurons are surrounded by inhibitory GABA neurons. In the latter, not all transcriptional systems pull in the same direction. For example, while gene expression associated with adrenergic and dopamin-ergic actions would clearly heighten arousal, expression of the gene for prostaglandin-D synthase (promoting sleep) or opioid receptors would have the opposite effect. All control systems – biologic, electronic, or digital – face similar requirements for balance among activating and suppressive subsystems, within the limitations of the overall system.

Wide ranges of temporal and spatial properties. Different neurons within arousal sys-tems have different time constants with respect to the regulation of their electrical activity. Consider the fastest mechanisms for spreading electrical excitation – gap junctions, also called "electrical synapses." Some neurons in the hindbrain reticular formation express the gene that codes for Connexin-36, the protein through which electrically charged molecules can travel rapidly from one nerve cell to an adjacent nerve cell (Martin et al., 2011). Then, of course, there are regular, chemical synapses, operating on time scales of milliseconds. But some hindbrain reticular neurons likely respond to very slow-changing signals, since we have preliminary evidence that a few of such neurons lie outside the blood–brain barrier and, indeed, as mentioned above and detailed in Chapter 2, Inna Tabansky et al. (2018) has discovered large medullary reticular ("Nucleus GigantoCellularis," NGC) neurons with molecular and morphologic properties that support intimate relations with blood vessels, potential "chemosensors." Chemical signals from the blood certainly will fluctuate with much slower time courses than electrical signals among neurons.

How this wide range of temporal properties is used in the CNS in an adaptive fashion is not clear. Do arousal-related neuronal changes have to occur in certain order? I think of the NGC neurons in the medullary reticular formation as "first responders," but that sup-position simply is inferred from what we know about them (Chapter 2). Is there a hierar-chy amongst different components of arousal responses? If so, to what extent do different aspects of brain arousal have to be synchronized? Or are there ideal delays amongst sub-systems? With respect to the human brain, are subsystem parameters optimized in the normal case, or is there room for improvement? Are alterations in timing a potential cause of the types of maladies listed below? All of these questions need answers.

This uncertainty also prevails for the range of spatial properties of arousal-related neu-rons. Again, are they optimized in the normal human brain, or could they be improved? Chapters 2 through 6 present the idea of modularity within the overall A/P, L system that governs arousal, with different modules theoretically contributing different properties and characteristics to the overall system. Classically, non-neuroscientists theorizing the nervous system began with random systems, but that approach almost certainly is wrong. Instead, considering the medullary reticular formation, for example, we have very large glutamatergic neurons whose axons travel long distances (Jones and Yang, 1985; Jones, 2003; Martin et al., 2011; Tabansky et al., 2018) surrounded by small, inhibitory GABA neurons, presumably to keep the big cells under control (see Chapter 2). Alberto Barabási (2009), Jeong et al. (2000), and their colleagues have conceived of systems in which a very few of highly interconnected nodes linked by a small number of long-distance lines are surrounded by large numbers of local units. We do not know, yet, the extent to which his thinking will help us finish analyzing CNS arousal systems.

Assays of Generalized CNS Arousal

Setting up an assay that measures the components of the operational definition (above) of arousal in experimental laboratory animals is relatively easy. The idea was to get total control over the environment of each mouse, housed singly (Garey et al., 2003; Weil et al., 2010; Proekt et al., 2012). Thus, each experimental chamber containing our generalized arousal assay had a mouse housed with no stimuli coming from the outside world. The operational definition of GA has three parts: motoric, sensory, and emotional. *Motoric*: we measure every movement each mouse makes, with 20 millisecond time resolution, 24 hours per day, and 7 days per week. *Sensory*: we used three sensory modalities that could be applied without intruding into the assay chamber and which have three different neuroanatomical sensory pathways: odor through the olfactory nerves, light touch through the dorsal roots of the spinal cord, and vestibular through the eighth cranial nerve. *Emotion*: to achieve a measurement that could validly be called emotion, we chose fear. With electrical shock to the feet, we could establish conditioned fear to which individual mice would be more or less reactive. We have used this assay to breed animals for high arousal and low arousal (see below), and are now following animals across the state transition from the light part of the light cycle (low arousal) to the dark part (high arousal).

For human subjects and patients, three circumstances in life demand arousal measurements and each contains its own "zero condition" or "null state:" disorders of consciousness, in which the lowest condition is coma; sleep, in which deepest sleep has its own physiological properties; and anesthesia, in which depth of anesthetization, e.g., during surgery, requires exquisitely sensitive measurement (see Chapter 8).

Coma: Historically, the most widely used behavioral measurement was formulated as the Glasgow Coma Scale, recently modified as the Glasgow-Liege Scale. The methodology of measurement is crucial for guiding treatment of patients who have some chance of recovery through the vegetative state to normal consciousness (Giacino et al., 2012).

The Glasgow Coma Scale rates the patient from 1 (the worst condition) to 6 (the best). The number is based on three types of observations. First, the Eye: from the lowest (does not open eyes) to the highest (opens eyes spontaneously). Second, Verbal: from the lowest (makes no sounds or only incomprehensible sounds) to the highest (well oriented and conversing normally). Finally, Motor: at worst, the patient makes no movements or only makes a reflex withdrawal from a painful stimulus. At best, the patient can make voluntary movements in response to commands.

In Professor Nicholas Schiff's efforts to bring formerly comatose vegetative state patients to a higher state of functional recovery, two types of innovation are included. First, high-end vegetative-state patients – patients who have shown sporadic ability to communicate – are chosen for further study. Second, a revised measurement scale is used (Giacino et al., 2012, Table 1). Not only are arousal, attention, and the ability to hear measured in the normal way, but there is also emphasis on the ability to follow commands. This brings in a higher degree of motor control and language comprehension and linguistic communication.

Sleep. From a physiological point of view, assays of sleep stages can emphasize either behavioral or electrical properties. Learning from Mountcastle (1974, pp. 261–2), behaviorally one looks for "elevation of thresholds for many reflexes," reduction in muscle tone, flaccid limbs, narrow pupils, and a decrease in peripheral autonomic sympathetic activity. In terms of cortical electrical activity (EEG), changes proceed from the high frequency waves (20 Hz or higher per second) of an awake, alert patient through intermediate stages to the deepest sleep occasioned by the slowest EEG waves – so-called delta waves of about 1 to 4 per second. Disorders of sleep include difficulty in getting to sleep, fragmented sleep, hypersomnia, and waking up too early (Weitzman, 1981).

Anesthesia. One of the three "null states" of CNS arousal is deep anesthesia. See Stanski and Shafer (2005): Modern measurements of the anesthetic state depend on at least six components – responses to incoming stimuli, ability to mount motor responses, concentrations of analgesic components (pain killers), concentrations of hypnotic components (which promote sleep-like states), concentrations of other relevant drugs like muscle relaxants, and the interactions among these components (from Stanski, 2005, Table 31.1). It is recognized that different components among these six operate at different levels of the neuraxis. EG local anesthetics work on peripheral nerves; there are spinal-acting opioids; other drugs work in the brainstem; and hypnotics are thought to work in the cerebral cortex. As a result of increasing anesthetic depth, for example, the patient's responses to calling his name, light touch, shouting, pinprick, and finally stronger painful stimuli as would result from the incision decreases. The ease with which appropriate anesthetic depth is reached depends on a large number of physiological factors, including, for example, pregnancy, thyroid gland status, and the duration over which the patient has been anesthetized. As far as the electroencephalography is concerned, anesthesiologists and neurologists have developed a complex measurement called the Bispectral Index. When this index is near 100, the EEG is dominated by small-amplitude high-frequency waves. The patient is awake and his memory intact. For general anesthesia, which is surgery-appropriate, the Index is in the neighborhood of 50 or 60. EEG waves are at low frequencies, large in amplitude. Some of these features depend on what part of the cortex is being recorded. When the Index is zero, the cortex electrical scene is silent in the so-called isoelectric state. Besides the straightforward electroencephalogram, neurologists can use the measurements of sensory-evoked cortical responses to electrical, auditory, or visual stimuli. The simplest summary is that one expects anesthesia to cause decreased amplitudes and increased latency of evoked responses (e.g., Figures 38.13–38.15 in Miller, 2005).

Recovery from anesthesia is just as interesting to study as the induction of the anesthetic state. At first one might think that the cerebral cortex would recover in a smooth, monotonic curve, following the gradual lowering of anesthetic level. That turns out not to be true. Knowing that, it was not clear how, after a large perturbation, the anesthetized brain explores the vast space of potential neuronal activity states to recover those compatible with consciousness. My lab analyzed EEG recovery from deep anesthesia to show that neuronal activity *en route* to consciousness is confined to a low-dimensional "subspace" (Hudson et al., 2014). That is, in this subspace, neuronal activity forms discrete metastable states persistent on a scale of minutes. The network of transitions that links these metastable states is structured such that some states form hubs that connect groups of otherwise disconnected states. Although many paths through the network are possible, in order to ultimately enter the activity state compatible with consciousness the brain must first pass through these hubs in an orderly fashion. The physiological interpretations of these hubs remain to be discovered.

Cardiovascular monitoring is important for the proper regulation of anesthesia. Heart rate and arterial blood pressure measures are standard. The anesthesiologist expects a lowered heart rate but still high enough to avoid dangerous bradycardia. Blood pressure is lowered, but its measurement may be complicated if there is pain. Of course, respiratory monitoring is important as well. While to the layman respiratory frequency and depth would be obvious measurements, the relevant measurements for the anesthesiologist concentrate on blood gasses: "the addition of O_2 to blood and the elimination of CO_2," (Miller, 2005, p. 1438). Finally, body temperature can be expected to fall during anesthesia, if only as a consequence of cardiovascular changes.

Interim summary

In an effort to reframe thinking about changes in states of arousal of brain and behavior, this book offers the concept of "generalized CNS arousal" (GA), a primitive undifferentiated force deeper than and fundamental to the usual motivational states (sex, hunger, etc.). This chapter gives GA an operational definition and has listed its operating requirements. GA is crucial for all cognitive functions and essential for normal emotional expression. While neuroscientists measure GA in laboratory mice, medical doctors effectively track GA in the fields of disorders of consciousness, sleep, and anesthesiology.

Evidence for the Existence of GA

At this point, the chapter has provided a concept of generalized CNS arousal, an operational definition, operating requirements, a sense of its importance, and measurements appropriate for laboratory animals and human patients. But is it possible to prove that GA actually exists? Four lines of evidence offer proof: psychological, genetic, statistical, and mechanistic. This section covers these starting with the oldest evidence.

Psychology. The oldest line of evidence for the existence of a brain function called "generalized arousal" came from psychologists who study normal human behavior and personality. In psychology, the story of arousal started with the famous Harvard philosopher and psychologist William James (1890). He coupled arousal with bodily changes and called it one of the "coarser emotions" (p. 449) and, in the manner of differential psychology, targeted it as contributing to individual differences in temperament (p. 475). After James, a twentieth-century tradition began analyzing human personality, led by Gordon Allport at Harvard. In that tradition, a professor of psychology at the University of North Carolina, Elizabeth Duffy (1962), treated "activation" as a central concept in the regulation of behavior. While she considered activation to depend on "the extent of release of potential energy, stored in the tissues of the organism, as this is shown in activity or response" (p. 17), her use of the concept essentially anticipates my approach to generalized CNS arousal. In fact, on p. 19 she says it is "possible to define activation as the arousal which occurs in the absence of physical exertion or the arousal found when we subtract from measures of activation the effects of physical activity." Consequences of high levels of such arousal would include heightened sensory sensitivity and faster, stronger responses.

Likewise, the experimental psychologist at Brown University, the prolific Harold Schlosberg, used the "level of activation," obviously arousal, as one of his "three dimensions of emotion" (Schlosbeg, 1954, see Figure 1).

Other examples came from psychologists who incorporated neurophysiology into their work. For instance, Donald Hebb (1955) used "generalized activation" as part of his psychological theory of motivation to account for the vigor of motivated behavior. The most graphic result of this behavioral thinking yielded the "circumplex" theory of personality (Russell, 1980; Posner et al., 2005). For this kind of picture, a circle is drawn and then two diametric lines are drawn at 90 degree angles to each other. One of those diameters labels the valence of a person's temperament: sunny to the right, negative to the left. The other diameter displays the generalized arousal dimension, high and forceful at the top, weak and timid at the bottom.

James Russell, a statistically inclined professor of psychology at Boston College, has considered many ways of measuring emotion with special attention to how different emotions relate to each other. The most solid results (Russell, 1980) came when various features of emotion were plotted on and within a theoretical circle in which the 90 degree point was labeled "arousal" and at 270 degrees, at the other end of that diameter, sleepiness. In terms of the frequencies with which it was given the primary designation on the circular scheme, it was always number one. More generally, various studies by psychologists over a period of 20 years *always* featured a major dimension: high arousal versus low arousal. In Russell's words, as he related the positive and negative valence of feelings to arousal "While in general arousal increases with positive or negative valence (a so-called V-shaped relation), there are large differences among individuals in how these two fundamental dimensions of affect are related in people's experience." (Kuppens et al., 2016). Russell's team reported that the steepness of the V-shaped relation between valence and arousal increases with extraversion within cultures, and that between eastern and western cultures significant difference in steepness could be discerned. From the point of view of this book, the most important finding was the robustness of the generalized arousal concept in personality theory.

Likewise, Rowe and Plomin (1977) took the structure of temperament that they had earlier proposed, which included an arousal-like dimension, and compared it to their more recent data. The arousal-like dimension, named "attention span-persistence," continued to be supported as existing in a significant manner.

While these personality characterizations were going on in the Americas, European biologists were following a parallel, but more naturalistic, path to the generalized arousal concept. Instead of studying humans in laboratories and hospitals, these biologists tended to observe animals in the animals' own habitat. For example, the Nobel prize-winning German ethologist Konrad Lorenz used a generalized arousal-like concept to explain "variations in intensity in the performance of instinctive responses," and relied on the magnitude of a global arousal force to do that (Lorenz, 1965). The behavioral biology textbook author Eibl-Eibesfeldt (1970) used generalized arousal to account for "a general motor restlessness and the expression of a specific readiness to act."

Some of the work on human arousal takes a developmental point of view. Harvard's Jerome Kagan was a leader in this field. Kagan and Snidman (1999) reported that a certain percentage of children are "born with a temperamental bias that predisposes them to be highly reactive to unfamiliar stimulation as infants and to be fearful of or avoidant to unfamiliar events and people as young children." They have "more reactive cardiovascular system, asymmetry of cortical activation in EEG favoring a more active right frontal area, more power in the EEG in the higher frequency range." This temperamental bias is contrasted with its opposite: "a consistently fearless and spontaneous profile." Overall,

Kagan's data pointed toward a developmental stability of personality in the arousal dimension. Children designated as "high reactive" or "low reactive" at a very early age tended to show those same personality features as young adults.

Other personality studies proceeded in a framework of clinical psychology. Here, generalized arousal as a concept found its home in H. J. Eysenck's studies of extraversion (Eysenck and Eysenck, 1967). For him, extraversion comprised a dimension of every person's temperament. High arousal would characterize introverts looking to ramp down social stimulation. Extroverts would display as the opposite.

In more recent times, it is hardly surprising that behavioral evidence for generalized arousal took a genetic turn. C.R. Cloninger is a genetically trained psychiatrist at Washington University of St. Louis School of Medicine. Generalized arousal was encased in his approaches to personality based in genetics, approaches that featured a "persistence" dimension defined as "persevering, ambitious (vs. easily discouraged), overachieving, etc.. In Stallings et al. (1996), Cloninger's model of temperament, including "persistence," received confirmation. Interestingly, a four-dimensional genetic factor structure was required to match temperamental genetic analyses for women, while for men only three genetic factors were necessary to explain the genetic variance among temperamental dimensions. Exactly what these genetic "factors" are remain unclear. To my knowledge nobody has tried to conceive exactly how a certain pattern of gene expression would lead to the personality structures these psychologists and psychiatrists have defined.

The autonomic nervous system's contributions to generalized arousal are obvious. Rooted in the classical physiological studies of Walter Cannon, one hundred years ago, the delicate interplay between the detailed neurochemistry and molecular biology of autonomic (sympathetic, for exciting cardiovascular and other systems, and parasympathetic, for quieting them down) neurons and psychological state has been pushed forward by Julian Thayer (Hagemann et al., 2003; Smith et al., 2017), in the department of psychiatry at the University of Arizona. Thayer's main concern has been to discover neural networks in the brain that regulate and coordinate autonomic responses. As he sees it, "numerous cortical and subcortical regions show co-occurring activity with autonomic nervous system responses in emotion." A variety of different basic emotions share common autonomic concomitants, which are linked to the arousal dimension of emotion.

More recently, Trofimova and Robbins (2016) recognized "the unidimensional construct of General Arousal as utilised by models of temperament in differential psychology" for example, to underlie "Extraversion." These authors understand that twentieth-century psychologists needed some kind of generalized arousal dimension to account for their observations. They prefer, however, to address three complementary sub-forms of arousal based on the neurochemistry of three different monoaminergic signaling systems in the brain. My emphasis on a primitive, fundamental, elemental GA, and their more specific sources of arousal can be reconciled. At the end of the chapter, I will present a differential equation (1.1) which has GA as a major term on the right side of the equation, and more specific forms of arousal as other terms among many. The constants attached to each term vary across individuals and across time.

Here is the main point. Over many decades, large numbers of psychologists and psychiatrists have analyzed how human personalities and temperaments are put together. Biologists have as well. All of these have taken various approaches: highly statistical, clinical, genetic, autonomic physiology. But each approach needed an important dimension, one which I call generalized arousal (to distinguish GA from simple sexual arousal, hunger, thirst, fear, etc.) to explain their data.

Genetics. You cannot have genes for a brain function that does not exist. The newest evidence for GA comes from genetics, as summarized by Calderon et al. (2016). During the past 20 years, evidence for genetic contributions to GA has burgeoned. Clearly, large numbers of genes and their products contribute to the modification of GA and therefore to its existence. First, hypocretin is a GA chemical *par excellence*. Second, gene knockout studies show examples of other compounds contributing to GA. Thirdly, we can breed for GA, thus proving its existence.

Before launching into the three approaches, a clear perspective: a neurochemical and molecular consideration shows that each and every neurotransmitter or neuropeptide contributing to activity changes in GA pathways depends on at least four classes of genes for its proper regulation:

i. Genes for synthetic enzymes that produce the neurotransmitter or neuropeptide in the first place. At a minimum, genes encoding for norepinephrine, glutamate, acetylcholine, dopamine, and histamine are involved as all these neurotransmitters contribute to GA, in addition to the more recently discovered hypocretin/orexin gene.

ii. Genes for the corresponding receptors.

iii. Genes encoding transporters, proteins responsible for re-uptake of the neurotransmitter or neuropeptide back into the presynaptic ending.

iv. Genes encoding catabolic enzymes for breaking down the transmitter or peptide in a regulated manner.

As noted, three types of studies have resulted in large numbers of papers, and that number is growing quickly. In the first type of study, molecular geneticists clone and analyze genes with GA in mind. In the second type, gene products of interest for various type of behaviors are manipulated and changes in GA result. Thirdly, over a period of years, a team in my lab has managed to breed for high GA and low GA mice, a formal proof of the existence of GA that simply extended what we already knew from the breeding of dogs and horses.

A perfect example of the *first* approach is the gene for hypocretin (reviewed, Li et al., 2016), expressed in about 3000 neurons in a very restricted portion of the lateral hypothalamus. Cloning of this gene was reported by the lab of Luis de Lecea in 1998, and was also cloned and called "orexin" by the Yanagisawa lab in Tsukuba, Japan. Two features of the hypocretin gene products qualify it for roles that serve generalized arousal. First, manipulating the gene shows clearly that it regulates, in de Lecea's words, "the boundaries and transitions between sleep and wakefulness." Second, axons projecting from hypocretin neurons project widely, ascending toward the forebrain and descending to the hindbrain. In fact, my lab has shown orexin receptor genes expressed in giant neurons in the medulla, just above the spinal cord (Martin et al., 2011; Tabansky et al., 2018). One interpretation of the biological function of hypocretin is that it fosters wakefulness under conditions that both seeking food and food intake are necessary to restore proper energy balance (Yamanaka et al., 2003).

Optogenetic activation of hypocretin neurons can wake up mice from sleep (Adamantidis et al., 2007). Conversely, optogenetic silencing of hypocretin neurons can induce sleep during the light phase of the daily light cycle (Tsunematsu et al., 2011).

Part of the power of the hypocretins in preserving wakefulness seems, in part, to lie in their ability to work through classical monoaminergic systems that serve arousal. These include noradrenergic neurons, since hypocretin axons project to the noradrenergic source in the hindbrain, the locus coeruleus. Another monoamine system affected is dopamine (emanating from the ventral tegmental area). Also, histamine (produced in the tuberomammillary nucleus in the medial hypothalamus. Serotonin, as well (produced in neurons in the raphe neurons on the midline of the midbrain). Importantly, hypocretin neurons project into the large cholinergic neurons of the basal forebrain, neurons which are important for waking activity in the cerebral cortex. Here I cite more detail regarding these five hypocretin targets, in order.

Matt Carter, in the de Lecea lab focused on the relationship between hypocretin output from the hypothalamus and the adrenergic neurons of locus coeruleus. In 2010, the de Lecea lab reported that "there is a frequency-dependent, causal relationship among locus coeruleus firing, cortical activity, sleep-to-wake transitions and general locomotor arousal." Then (2012) they used a new technique called optogenetics to selectively inhibit locus coeruleus neurons during hypocretin stimulation, and as a result blocked hypocretin-mediated sleep-to-wake transitions. Carter et al. (2013), now at the University of Washington, reviewed this work and reflected on how hypocretin neurons, which receive inputs from wide-ranging regions of the brain, calibrate behavioral arousal levels appropriate to the organism's needs which, of course, change from time to time. Working through locus coeruleus, hypocretin signaling not only facilitates the sleep-to-wake transition but also helps to prevent the "fragmentation of sleep/wake states." Second, through the dopamine system, hypocretin neuron activation fosters preferences for stimuli associated with drug and food rewards. Thirdly, histaminergic neurons receive inputs from hypocretin cells and seem to work in parallel with hypocretin in promoting arousal. Fourth, through serotonergic systems hypocretin might affect sleep physiology (and its disorders). Finally, through cholinergic neurons in the basal forebrain, hypocretin seems to improve cognitive ability, as blocking hypocretin action there reduces performance in a task that required sustained attention.

A *second* approach to the genetics of arousal follows a different route to discovery. In the field of work just reviewed, the scientists cloned a gene involved in generalized CNS arousal and thus stimulated an entirely new field of work: describing neuroanatomical projections, discovering cognate receptors, analyzing mechanisms of action, and so forth. This second approach comes from gene knockout studies that were initiated for a different reason, and the arousal data were eventually discovered in later, follow-up studies. For example, the gene for estrogen receptor α (ERα) first garnered great interest because of its involvement in sex behaviors (Ogawa et al., 1998a, b). Later, Joan Garey (Garey et al., 2003) extended our behavioral analyses to include arousal measurements.

My lab wondered whether the genes for the cell nuclear receptors through which estrogens strongly drive female sex behaviors, could be involved in the more global brain function, generalized CNS arousal. We studied female mice, individually housed, sleeping in their home cages as they do during the light phase of the daily light cycle. We hoped that by doing the assays this way, we could remove imprecision due to ongoing activities, as well as biases relating to fear and anxiety, from the experimental protocol. The answers were clear.

For all sensory modalities tested, α-ER knockout (α-ERKO) female mice were less responsive to sensory stimuli than their WT female littermate controls. Surprisingly, disruption of the gene for the closely related ER-β, a likely gene duplication product, did not have the same effect. That is, α-ERKO female mice were less aroused by vestibular, tactile, olfactory, or auditory stimuli than their littermate WT controls. This result did not occur in β-ERKO females. Likewise, in terms of locomotor activity in running wheels, highest during the dark phase of the daily light cycle, α-ERKO females were less active. Interestingly, this phenotype depended on age; older α-ERKO females were subject to the genetic effect, whereas the younger α-ERKO females were not. Again, the differences between β-ERKO females and their WT littermate controls were not significant (data not shown). The graphs for running wheel activity of β-ERKO mice and their controls were virtually identical. In sum, α-ERKO females had less generalized arousal in that they were less responsive to external stimuli and less motorically active.

Other studies measuring motoric activity gave similar results. Spiteri et al. (2012) reported that reduction of the ER-α gene product specifically in the neurons of the medial preoptic area reduced movement. This finding replicated the work of Ogawa et al. (2003), who had also reported that gonadectomized αERKO female were significantly less active than αWT mice in open field tests, whereas beta-ERKO females tended to be more active than β-WT mice.

A *third* line of genetic evidence for generalized arousal is that you can breed for this function. You can't breed for a brain function that does not exist. Since we knew that we would be breeding mice for a multigenic function, we went for advice to behavior geneticist David Blizard, of Pennsylvania State University. He advised us to start with a strain of mice that had a high degree of genetic heterogeneity. This type of strain had indeed been achieved by Gardner Lindzey and Donald Thiessen many years before. The high genetic heterogeneity had resulted from an extensive intercross of more than eight outbred strains (and was called Het-8). As mentioned, our generalized arousal assay featured mice housed singly and cut off absolutely from the outside world. No sound, no vibration, no odors. Using a 12-hour lights-on and 12-hour lights-off daily cycle, we were measuring every movement each mouse made, with 20 millisecond time resolution, 24 hours per day, 7 days per week. Those measurements accounted for the Motoric part of the generalized arousal operational definition (see above).

For the sensory responsiveness aspect of the operational definition, my lab used three sensory modalities that could be applied without intruding into the assay chamber and which have three different neuroanatomical sensory pathways: odor through the olfactory nerves, light touch through the dorsal roots of the spinal cord, and vestibular through the eighth cranial nerve. Regarding the third and last part of the operational definition of generalized arousal (GA), emotional reactivity, what can we count on for emotion in a mouse? Fear, for sure. Therefore, using electrical shock to the feet, we could establish conditioned fear to which individual mice would be more or less reactive. Starting with "generation zero" of male and female mice we determined, using a combination of all three components of the operational definition – sensory, motor, and emotion – which displayed the highest GA and which the lowest. Then, of course, we mated highest GA males to highest GA females and low to low, to make the next generation of mice. We repeated this procedure generation after generation.

By the seventh generation, we were successful in establishing high and low GA genetic lines of mice, proving that it is possible to breed for GA and that GA must therefore exist (Weil et al., 2010). Further, there were implications for arousal-related behaviors. Animals defined as high-arousal animals by the assay exhibited greater levels of anxiety-like behavior, reduced exploratory behavior, and were more sexually excitable (Weil et al., 2010) in comparison with those defined as low arousal. The divergence of behaviors between the high GA line and the low GA line after the seventh generation offers independent evidence for the existence of GA.

Thus, we have developed a behavioral assay of generalized CNS arousal that takes into account the three proposed facets of arousal behavior: motor activity, sensory responsivity, and emotionality. Genetically heterogeneous mice were tested in this assay and rank orders were established for high and low arousal on each of the three subscales of generalized arousal. The mice that exhibited the highest (and lowest) scores summed across the three subscales in each generation were then used as the founders of the next generation. Generalized arousal measured by our assay was higher in mice from the high line. These data indicate that it is possible to generate, even within a few generations, divergent lines of mice exhibiting differential patterns of generalized arousal.

In a sense, our mouse breeding study extended in a formal, rigorous manner, what professional animal breeders already knew (reviewed, Ogawa et al., 2004; Calderon et al., 2016). In a large number of vertebrate species, genetic differences have been tied to differences in behaviors that require high CNS arousal, such as aggressive behaviors. Consider Siamese fighting fish, a large number of aggression differences in lines of mice, different strains of rats that have been selected for attack latencies, and breeds of dogs such as pit bulls and rottweilers.

In fact, because of the ease of observation of temperamental differences in dogs, the book Genetics and the Social Behavior of the Dog (1965) by Scott and Fuller became a classic in the field of behavioral genetics. Further evidence is derived from the breeding of dogs from wolves. As reviewed (Ogawa et al., 2004; Calderon et al., 2016) the domestication of dogs started approximately 30,000 years ago, and the very existence of domesticated dogs (which emerged about 15,000 years ago in East Asia) indicates that genetic factors contribute to arousal-dependent behaviors, and are thus implicated in GA. Domestication involved animals being selected for specific behavioral traits, and this has resulted in many different dog strains with very different behavioral profiles. For example, the cocker spaniel and Shetland sheepdog have much lower behavioral reactivity to startling stimuli than the beagle, basenji, or wire-haired fox terrier (Scott and Fuller, 1965).

Even horses have different temperaments. A high GA horse, perhaps a racing thoroughbred, will be walked onto the track with a low GA horse who maintains calm behavior in the dyad. This makes them more (or less) susceptible to provocations leading to fighting. Similarly, horses can be bred for specific behavioral characteristics; as noted, the rapid responsivity of the thoroughbred race horse (high) GA compared to the calm and unresponsiveness of the horse to which it is tethered (low GA) for behavioral management in loud, unpredictable environments.

Back in the laboratory, in a breeding study involving rats, animals were bred for low GA (here defined as tameness and tolerance to human presence and interaction). Derived from wild rats, tame ones were selected for 32 years. This group expressed less aggression, fear, or defensive behaviors compared to controls (not tamed) in 11 out of 13 components scored in the behavior of rats toward a human hand. They were also more exploratory and exhibited fewer anxiety-like behaviors. Interestingly, these behaviors were associated with smaller adrenal glands, lower levels of corticosterone and serotonin in serum. In addition, cross-fostering experiments, as reviewed (Calderon et al., 2016), showed that these behavioral results were not related to maternal care suggesting that the behavioral differences observed between the lines have a genetic basis. Albert et al. mapped the locations of DNA sequence differences that contributed to differences between the tame and aggressive rat lines (Albert et al., 2009). More recently, they also identified, using messenger RNA sequencing and a DNA mapping method, multiple genes influenced by the genetic variants from the tame and aggressive lines (Heyne et al., 2014). Candidate genes that may play a causal role in these behaviors have been implicated in anxiety and stress, both related to GA.

Statistics. The impact of GA on behavior was revealed by using principal component analysis (PCA) in a set of five populations of ovariectomized mice described in detail in Garey et al. (2003), Morgan and Pfaff (2001), and Frohlich et al. (2001, 2002). That is, in preparation for evaluating hormone effects and hormone receptor gene influences on fundamental processes of behavioral arousal, we subjected 48 ovariectomized female mice to a rigid protocol of several tests bearing on arousal concepts (Frohlich et al., 2001). The central hypothesis was that results would organize themselves according to capacities for sensory alertness, motor activity, and emotional reactivity. The large table of across-mouse correlations was subjected to factor analysis and cluster analysis. Results provided evidence for a general arousal (one-factor solution) which, however, accounted for only 29.72 percent of the variance. Then, we (Frohlich et al., 2002) investigated the roles of thyroid hormone and estradiol in altering the statistical structure of arousal measures. Factor and cluster analysis indicated the statistical structure of arousal measures to be reasonably robust across hormonal conditions. Hormone effects on arousal components are of interest because of their likely contributions to emotional states and cognitive performance.

Later, mice were subjected to our high throughput assay, described above, that quantitatively measured: (i) motor activity: distance traveled, total movement duration, and voluntary movement in a running wheel; (ii) sensory responses to external stimuli: auditory, vestibular, tactile, and olfactory stimuli; and (iii) emotional reactivity: motor activity and freezing behavior in a conditioned fear paradigm (Garey et al., 2003; Weil et al., 2010). These variables were weighted by their contribution to the explanation of the variance. Despite multiple experimental variables such as experimental design and mice populations, the covariance analysis of various arousal-related response measures reported that GA accounted for between 29 percent and 45 percent of the variance in behavioral results across the studies. GA accounts for significantly more real data than in any random-number control.

Likewise, nothing similar to the GA factor appeared in control data sets in which data entries were scrambled. That is, in all experiments reanalyzed by PCA, generalized arousal accounted for a significant amount of the data (about one-third), with the lowest contribution at 29.7 percent and the highest at 45 percent. Surprisingly, this range held true despite (i) different populations of mice, (ii) different investigators, (iii) different experimental manipulations and details of response measures, and (iv) different configurations of individual, particular factor analysis solutions involving four to six factors for each experiment. The one-factor solution was robust, shown in three ways: (i) it was never identical to the first factor of a particular multifactor analysis. Indeed, it was, as might be expected, correlated, but that correlation was always significantly <1.0 ($P < 0.001$); (ii) it accounted for significantly more data than in a random-number control; and (iii) it accounted for significantly more data than in a control in which marginal averages were held constant but the individual data entries were scrambled randomly. All of these arguments indicate that the mathematical structure of arousal includes a primitive, undifferentiated form that accounts for about one-third of the data in female mice.

As summarized by Calderon et al. (2016), the other contributions to arousal – for example due to thirst, hunger, fear, anger, and other motivators – would all be expected to account for some of the variance and are reflected in the differential equation written below (1.1). Thus, in quantitative terms, if behavioral arousal were viewed as a differential equation (see below) with many different types of arousal represented by many independent terms, the GA term would be large and significant, but would account for less than half the variance, compared with the sum of all the other terms (e.g., arousal due to hunger, thirst, or fear, and perhaps other terms not yet named). In sum, the statistics of principal components analysis support the conclusion that GA exists, but also indicates the importance of other, specific forms of arousal.

Brain mechanisms. You can't have mechanisms for a function that does not exist. Long ago, neurophysiologists Dempsey and Morison (1942a, b) and Moruzzi and Magoun (1949) revealed effects of brainstem stimulation that were read out in terms of electrical recordings from the cortex. For a long time, these reports did not lead anywhere. In the case of Dempsey/Morison, the large number of medical scientists serving in World War II was a factor. In the Moruzzi/Magoun case, the fascination of neurophysiologists with specific sensory and motor systems distracted them from matters related to arousal. Thus, David Hubel and Torsten Wiesel won the Nobel Prize for studies of the visual cortex and Sir John Eccles won for studies of motor neurons.

Nevertheless, during the last thirty years or so, the neurobiological mechanisms for changes of state of the entire CNS – the exact opposite of specific sensory systems – have "caught up" enough to merit this book-length treatment. An example would be the neuroanatomical summary of reticular formation morphology by the McGill University neurobiologist Barbara Jones (Jones, 2003).

Thus additional evidence for the *existence* of GA lies in the fact that we know a lot about *how GA works*. Chapters 2 through 6 march up the neuraxis from the "master cells" for GA in the medullary reticular formation through the pons, the midbrain, the hypothalamus, and the central thalamus. Chapter 7 shows how GA contributes to behaviors that depend on high-arousal states – behaviors such as sex, fear, and aggression. Conversely, Chapter 8 explains low-arousal conditions like coma, deep sleep and deep anesthesia. All of these chapters will spin out evidence that GA exists; it is alive and well in the mammalian brain.

With four independent lines of evidence for the existence of GA – psychological, genetic, statistical, and mechanistic – we felt comfortable theorizing about GA as a physical process. It turns out that flipping from a not-aroused state appears to have the property of a physical phase transition (Pfaff and Banavar, 2007), and should demonstrate the "scaling" and accompanied "power law behavior" – behavior governed by a simple exponential equation (see Equation 10.1) that produces the same dynamics from tiny scales to huge scales. In our laboratory mice this prediction proves true so far, and I suspect that this type of transition is universal among vertebrates.

Physical, Quantitative Properties of GA

Pursuing our determination to think about arousal systems with a precision typical of the physical sciences, we turned to Penn State professor of physics, Jayanth Banavar (now at Oregon), a friend from my many visits to that campus and a master of the art of clear explanation. We knew that we needed to generate a systematic set of hypotheses about the regulation of generalized CNS arousal as a function that bears on virtually all aspects of human and animal behavior. Our ideas were expected to apply universally among vertebrates. We started with the idea that when rapid changes of state of the CNS would be required – for example when a rapid response to a stimulus would be important to achieve – that *linear* dynamics in generalized arousal mechanisms would *not* be sufficient. Nonlinear dynamics, as found in chaotic systems, could provide tremendous amplification of CNS arousal signals and would also confer exquisite sensitivity to the initial state of the system. The hypothesis, therefore, that in the not-aroused state chaotic dynamics prevail, is very attractive because they are deterministic and because they link the elegant mathematics of chaos to the concept of a fundamental property of the vertebrate CNS. But for coordinated movements as part of the behaviors thus initiated the system will have to emerge from chaos. Our second idea was that as neural systems pass from the chaotic non-aroused state to aroused states they pass through a classically defined phase transition. With the behavioral response activated, orderly movement control neurophysiology takes over (Pfaff and Banavar, 2007).

To understand our theory clearly, consider the analogy to a classical physical example of a phase transition, the liquid crystal. Arousal systems in the not-aroused or low-aroused animal are in a chaotic state. The controlled-chaotic state of Ott et al. (1994) would be perfectly appropriate. When the animal is sufficiently stimulated, the non-linear dynamics of deterministic chaos provide exponential amplification so that CNS systems can initiate orderly movement in response. By analogy to the liquid crystal, the disordered molecules at a higher temperature go through a phase transition to the ordered, crystalline state.

Experimental scientists are beginning to think along these lines, and some evidence for our theory has accrued. Bassett et al. (2006) obtained magnetoencephalographics from human subjects who were preforming a finger-tapping task. They used a variety of mathematical approaches to analyze several spectral domains in the subjects' cerebral cortical activity. The results showing the degree of synchronizability of this activity demonstrated, in their words, that "the brain networks are located dynamically on a critical point of the order/disorder transition." That is, their networks were close to the threshold of order/disorder transformation in all frequency bands, just like our theoretical liquid crystal analogy.

Another example of the importance of thinking about chaotic dynamics in relation to neural activity comes from findings in auditory neurophysiology. Certain nonlinear equations (e.g., 6.1) yielding chaotic dynamics demonstrate instabilities at fixed, special values of some given system parameter called "Hopf bifurcations." Marcelo Magnasco and his colleagues (2003) have presented evidence that the tuning curves of the cochlea in the auditory system are partly shaped by a set of mechanosensors poised precisely at the threshold of a Hopf instability. This application of nonlinearity in hearing achieves the advantages of a high degree of amplification and a sharp tuning curve even at low input intensity.

Magnasco and his colleagues have extended their evidence for "dynamic criticality" to the electrical activity of the human cerebral cortex (Alonso et al., 2014; Solovey et al., 2015). Dynamic criticality refers to "systems that persist at the boundary between stability and instability" and is typified by "systems highly susceptible to small external perturbations." Alonso et al. argue, and I agree, that we need neural mechanisms to constitute "an extended dynamical system that is close to a critical point and will neither decay nor explode, thus allowing for long range communication across the entire system." This type of system is just what we need, theoretically, to create a generalized CNS arousal system that protects us from dangers in the external world.

Alex Proekt, a medical doctor and neurophysiologist formerly in my lab, now at the University of Pennsylvania Medical School, noticed that the timing of many diverse behaviors from human communication to animal foraging form complex self-similar temporal patterns reproduced on multiple time scales. We envisioned and demonstrated a general framework for understanding how such scale invariance may arise in nonequilibrium systems, including those that regulate mammalian behaviors. In the following, we demonstrate that the predictions of this framework are in agreement with the detailed analysis of spontaneous mouse behavior observed in a simple unchanging environment. Analyses revealed that the specifics of the distribution of resources or competition among several tasks are not essential for the expression of scale-free dynamics. Importantly, we show that scale invariance observed in the dynamics of behavior can arise from the dynamics *intrinsic to the brain* (Proekt et al. 2012).

In physical systems, one observes scale invariance – a repetition of shape and dynamics from tiny physical scales through huge physical scales – near a critical point, for example, where water turns into steam or where the unaroused animal can become aroused. It has been suggested that the presence of power laws, defined above, in diverse living systems might imply that biological systems are poised in the vicinity of a continuous phase transitions. There are, however, fundamental differences between scale invariance exhibited by biological and physical systems. Criticality – the supersensitive responses to small stimuli – is confined to a small region in parameter space, and it is not clear how diverse biological systems are fine-tuned to exhibit criticality. But critical systems in physics are at equilibrium, whereas most processes occurring in living systems including animal behavior are not in equilibrium.

Behavior is often conceived as serving a particular purpose or as a response to a specific stimulus. However, even in the relative absence of these phenomena, all animals including humans readily exhibit spontaneous behavior. Spontaneous activation of behavior is the simplest case of animal behavior because it avoids the complexities added by specific behavioral tasks, interactions among individuals, and the specifics of the structure of the environment. Understanding the dynamics of spontaneous behavior therefore is a prerequisite for understanding behavioral dynamics in more complex settings. This was the focus of our analysis (Proekt et al., 2012).

Proekt worked with Professor Banavar and mathematician Amos Maritan to analyze the fine structure of the movements of mice in the GA assay described above. Importantly, systems going through a phase transition behave according to simple exponential equations called "power laws." Plotted on log:log coordinates – both the X-axis of the graph and the Y-axis of the graphs are scaled logarithmically rather than linearly – such systems yield straight lines. In accordance with our theory, our mice, during the dark phase of the daily light cycle, demonstrated straight lines over three orders of magnitude (Figure 1.1). These results (Proekt et al., 2012) are consistent with our phase transition theory summarized above.

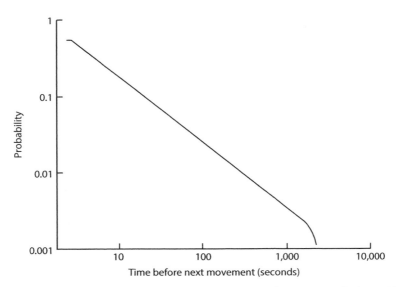

Figure 1.1 Sketch of the evidence from Proekt et al. (2012) that timing of the initiation of behavior follows a power law over three orders of magnitude. Such scale-free dynamics are typical of a phase transition. Results that are linear in a plot on log–log axes reveal power law dynamics.

Still working with the physicist Jayanth Banavar, we are now asking mathematical questions about the performance of laboratory mice as they go through the hypothesized phase transitions from the light part of the day (low CNS arousal) to the dark part (high CNS arousal) in a 12-hour light to 12-hour dark daily cycle. As we work with equipment that provides temporal resolution of 20 milliseconds, we ask, with the data from individual mice on individual days, what mathematical curves fit their activity change and what do equations suggest? How can we describe individual differences? Is the phase transition from high to low arousal the mirror image of the transition from low to high? Chapter 5 and equation 5.1 offer the first answers to these questions.

Maladies Due to Dysregulation of GA

There are many serious medical and public health problems resulting from failures of generalized CNS arousal. One obvious category is disorders of consciousness. While coma is mentioned here in Chapter 1, coma is, by definition, a temporary condition. Either the patient escapes from coma and enters a vegetative state or he dies. Vegetative state patients are not uniform in their range or severity of symptoms. Recently, there has been special attention given to "high end" vegetative-state patients – those who sporadically have shown some communication – because such patients may be responsive to treatments such as deep brain stimulation (Schiff et al., 2007). Stupor, as well, certainly involves arousal problems.

Another obvious patient group is that with mood disorders. All forms of depression would be included here but, among them, melancholic depression must reveal the most abnormal performance of GA mechanisms. Of course, the manic episodes of bipolar disorders represent GA mechanisms operating at dangerously high levels.

Consider the cognitive problems of some aging individuals and the apathy in some Alzheimer's patients. These have arousal components. Attention deficit hyperactivity disorder (ADHD) must feature periods of high motoric arousal, but ordinary neuroscientific thinking does not explain why Ritalin works when it does. In another context, I have hypothesized (2011) that autism spectrum disorders (ASD) depend, in part, on testosterone-enhanced arousal signals to the forebrain that result in a supersensitive amygdala.

In the working world, GA plays especially important roles in certain jobs that require high and sustained vigilance. The military is one example. It is said that even a trained sniper cannot maintain the necessary level of attention for longer than about 30 minutes. Shift work in which an individual rotates through two or three daily shifts takes its toll because of the challenge to the individual's circadian rhythms. Dangerous occupations like slicing meat or fish explode the size of the potential losses – e.g., decreased arousal resulting in even a moment of lapsed attention can cause the loss of a limb.

Public health failures like elevated lead concentration in drinking water can reduce cognitive performance through routes that include decreased GA. Perhaps the mysterious "fatigue states" are related. Thus some scientists think that they can follow certain environmental exposures that lead to Chronic Fatigue Syndrome, Fibromyalgia Syndrome, and Gulf War Syndrome. The first two are much more common among women and the third in men, but they all share many symptoms, one of which is decreased GA.

Some of the foregoing conditions are characterized by underperformance of GA mechanisms. But for some patients, *reducing* arousal level is necessary. Here are two examples. First, it is estimated that about 15 to 20 percent of American adults have sleep problems: some cannot get to sleep, while others have badly fragmented sleep or wake up too early. Secondly, anesthesia, as for surgery, is a highly sophisticated branch of medicine. The regulated reduction in arousal level was mentioned earlier in this chapter.

The beginning of this chapter portrayed generalized CNS arousal as fundamental to all cognitive abilities and essential for all emotional expressions, it could be possible to suppose that when arousal mechanisms are not working right there will be problems. This brief treatment supports that supposition.

Resolution of a Difference in Emphasis

As demonstrated, we have good evidence for a universal motivating "force" in the mammalian brain, an elementary set of mechanisms essential for the initiation of behavior. Other theorists would disagree. Trevor Robbins, for example, a distinguished behavioral biologist who is a professor at the University of Cambridge, portrays the "general arousal concept" as arising entirely from hypocretin neurons in the lateral hypothalamus (Trofimova and Robbins, 2016).

In a sense, Robbins' discomfort with the concept of generalized arousal dates back, in the history of psychology, to the opinions and work of Donald Broadbent, who led a prolific career in the Applied Psychology Unit of the Medical Research Council in Cambridge. Broadbent (1971) used the arousal concept in his work on vigilance (pp. 45–51) and recognized optimal levels of arousal (e.g., p. 48). But he also cited "difficulties in the concept of a single state of arousal" (pp. 440 and ff.). Briefly, the data from experiments featuring interactions between environmental conditions, including noise, sleepiness, time of day, and alcohol, could not be explained by a unitary concept of arousal.

Robbins prefers to emphasize noradrenalin (norepinephrine), dopaminergic, serotonergic, and cholinergic as having different arousal-related specialties. In his words, noradrenaline would be involved in the "expansion of alternatives," functions related to attention and orienting; dopaminergic neurons would be responsible for the "prioritizing of alternatives," matters related to the salience of individual stimuli; serotonin neurons responsible for "contextual" effects, the integration and maintenance of actions already begun; and acetylcholine neurons as having a "tonic" arousing influence. He argues that these subsystems interact! Thus, "first, there is likely no single neurotransmitter the release of which is independent of the action of other neurochemical systems, including other neurotransmitters. Monoaminergic (MA) systems regulate one another's release in a contingent manner via several mechanisms with different release patterns depending on the intensity of stimulation and the location and density of receptors" (Trofimova and Robbins, 2016). These two authors understand that the concept of generalized arousal is useful, as we document above, in clinical psychology. But they feel more comfortable emphasizing complementary sub-forms of arousal described briefly in the paragraph above.

Let us avoid a false dichotomy. Trevor Robbins much prefers to write about specific types of arousal states associated with particular transmitters (Trofimova and Robbins, 2016). I am impressed by the universality among vertebrates including humans of generalized arousal. Hope is not lost for an orderly approach to these questions. In my drive to render some parts of behavioral neuroscience amenable to mathematical treatment, I have imagined a differential equation that encompasses Robbins' approach as well as mine, to explain changes in overall arousal (A) as a function of time:

$$\frac{\partial A}{\partial t} = F(k_g A_g, k_h A_h, k_t A_t, k_f A_f, \ldots, k_n A_n) \tag{1.1}$$

where "g" denotes generalized arousal; "h," hunger; "t," thirst; "f," fear; and so forth.

This equation asserts that a component called GA plays a significant role in the overall arousal state of any vertebrate animal, including humans, but that other terms reflect obvious motivational influences on behavior, including sources of arousal yet to be identified.

We do not know the full number and identities of the terms in this equation, and we do not know how the terms comport with each other (probably not additive; perhaps multiplicative; sometimes exponential?). A long time ago, behavioral neuroscientists experimented on the relation of different bodily drive states to each other. For example, consider fear and sex. It has been reported that men looking at soft pornography considered the pictures sexier when they were balancing on tricky places from which they could fall, compared to men standing on a nice safe wide bridge. I have no doubt that molecular mechanisms for relations among terms in the equation above will emerge in coming years. Further, they will make biological sense because those relations evolved in a biologically adaptive manner.

Mathematical analogies. Thinking about GA mechanisms in physical and mathematical terms will lead to interesting things. Thus, Chapter 10 delves into classical Shannon information theory and modern network theory.

Summary

Thirteen years ago (leading to *Brain Arousal and Information Theory*) I proposed the concept of generalized CNS (central nervous system) arousal to reframe our theoretical approaches to the initiation of any vertebrate behavior. The book presented an operational definition of GA and listed GA's operating requirements. Quantitative assays for measuring GA are available for experimental animals and patients.

We now have years of new data on CNS arousal and a tremendous amount of new neurological work on disorders of consciousness. This book uses that data to reframe our thinking, to look at a vertically integrated, ladder-like A/P, L (L, standing both for longitudinal and ladder-like) network that produces GA.

Now we also have a theory that spells out a physical analogy for GA and presents the idea of the initiation of behavior as involving a physically defined phase transition. Moreover, we have mechanistic data that have led us to focus on large reticular formation nerve cells, NGC as the most powerful and essential neurons for initiating GA, the "master cells" for CNS arousal. Chapter 2 discusses those NGC neurons.

Chapter 10 delves into network theory in order to emphasize that, considering the largest reticular formation neurons – certainly including NGC (Chapter 2) – with tremendously large numbers of connections, and likewise considering the excess of small neurons with only local connections, we might be dealing with a scale-free GA system (Barabási, 2009; and for electrophysiological data, see He, 2014). If the largest reticular neurons are sending identical messages to a wide range of neuronal targets stretching from the lowest spinal cord to the thalamus and basal forebrain, *that is what integration means, taking many disparate signals and states and molding them to a singular initiative.*

The GA system achieves what network theorists call criticality, which includes the ability to make rapid and adaptive responses to tiny changes in inputs. Pfaff and Banavar (2007) theorized that such phase transitions characterize CNS arousal systems. Data from the Human Connectome Project subsequently have yielded evidence of scale-invariance (Taylor et al., 2017). A scale-free network can in principle lead to scale-free temporal behavior but is not logically or mathematically guaranteed to do so.

We could consider a rough analogy to information theory. Claude Shannon (1948) at Bell Labs came up with a simple equation (10.2) to summarize the amount of digital information flow *without any reference to the specific content or meaning of the message.* GA is the most prominent term in an equation (1.1) that accounts for the initiation of behavior *without any reference to the specific motivation connected with the behavior.*

Here I conjecture that major themes from the neuroscience literature in this book are actually related to each other. The A/P longitudinal, ladder-like signaling makes for high connectivity of GA systems and for the essence of "integration" by virtue of sending the same message to many different outlets. If this GA net is really scale-free, then certain scale-free features of GA-related behavior might be predicted. Further, I conjecture that the basic elements of GA systems are present universally in vertebrate brains.

Now, in the next chapter we'll address the medullary reticular formation with its giant neurons in NGC. The high "channel capacities" of these NGC neurons (due to multimodal inputs, widespread outputs, and high-frequency firing rates) fit well with the preceding paragraphs.

Giant Cells in the Medullary Reticular Formation

I have come to the view that the master cells for generalized CNS arousal (GA) are giant cells in the medullary reticular formation, neurons of the nucleus gigantocellularis (NGC). Moreover, if these are the origins of GA, then the "origins of the origins" can be spelled out in evolutionary, embryonic, and electrophysiological terms. This chapter will include these three points.

Historically, neurophysiologists related the brainstem to the electrical activity of the cerebral cortex by using both destructive intrusions and techniques of electrical stimulation. Early in the twentieth century, the Belgian neurologist Frederic Bremer made transections directly through the brainstem. When such a transection was at the level of the midbrain, the animal was stuck in a sleep-like state. In contrast, if the transection was at the bottom of the brainstem, the sleep–wake cycle was normal.

With respect to stimulation, Dempsey and Morison (1942a, b; Morison and Dempsey, 1942), reported that certain forms of electrical stimulation of the central thalamus over a long period of time recruited wave-like responses widely distributed in the electrical activity of the cerebral cortex. Later, Moruzzi and Magoun (1949) discovered that "direct stimulation of the brainstem core reproduced all the electrocortical features observed in the EEG arousal reaction associated with natural wakefulness" (reviewed Magoun, 1958, p. 77).

This chapter argues that certain large medullary neurons have the inputs, outputs, and genes properly expressed to serve as the "master neurons" for GA. These large medullary neurons are in the NGC of the medulla, just above the spinal cord (Figure 2.1). They have extensive inputs. They also have extensive outputs through axons ascending, and descending – and for some NGC neurons, *both* ascending and descending (Figure 2.2). In sum, they provide the essential driving force for elevating GA for entry into consciousness, for the initiation of behavior.

First it is important to highlight physiological properties of NGC neurons, followed by their morphological and genetic properties, so as to show that NGC neurons are capable of acting as "first responders," allowing the lab animal or human to respond to alarming and other salient stimuli.

Effects of Heightened Activity in NGC

My lab theorized that large neurons in the ventral and medial reticular formation of the medulla are critical for both autonomic and cortical arousal. To test this theory, we (Wu et al., 2007) anesthetized rats with urethane, lowered concentric bipolar stimulating

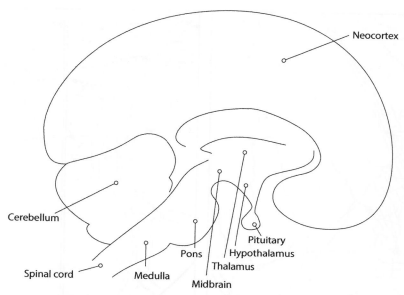

Neocortex

Cerebellum

Spinal cord

Medulla

Pons

Thalamus

Midbrain

Hypothalamus

Pituitary

Figure 2.1 A sketch of the human brain looking from the right side. Illustrated are embryological divisions of the brain: spinal cord, myencephalon (medulla), metencephalon (pons), mesencephalon (midbrain), diencephalon (thalamus and hypothalamus), and telencephalon (forebrain: neocortex). Not illustrated is the phylogenetically ancient forebrain, the "limbic system," which is tucked underneath the cortex

electrodes into the medullary reticular formation, and implanted electroencephalogram (EEG) and electrocardiogram (EKG) recording electrodes. We stimulated in the NGC region of the medullary reticular formation with pulse frequencies ranging from 50 to 300 Hz while recording cortical EEG and EKG. Electrical stimulation at either 200 or 300 Hz among the large medullary reticular neurons caused a significant reduction in the portion of the EEG power spectrum represented by delta-waves (0.1–4 Hz) and theta-waves (4.1–8 Hz). Correspondingly, there were increases in gamma-wave power (22–50 Hz), especially when using 300 Hz. Electrical stimulation also increased EKG. Controls against unanticipated spread of current spread (e.g., to the pyramidal tract) were three fold: (i) use of concentric bipolar electrodes, (ii) off-target controls not giving the same results, and (iii) no observed movement, as would have followed from pyramidal tract stimulation. Thus, electrical stimulation of the medial medullary reticular formation activates the cortical EEG even in deeply anesthetized animals, and also has an autonomic effect, higher frequency heart rate.

To confirm and extend the Wu et al. findings, a lab leader, medical doctor and neurophysiologist Diany Paola Calderon used a technique called optogenetics in deeply anesthetized mice (Calderon et al., 2018; see Figure 8.1). Optogenetics requires placing a light-sensitive protein at the specific location in the brain that you want to study. Some such light-sensitive proteins will cause the neuron in which they are placed to fire action potentials at a high frequency. Other such proteins have the opposite effect, inhibiting

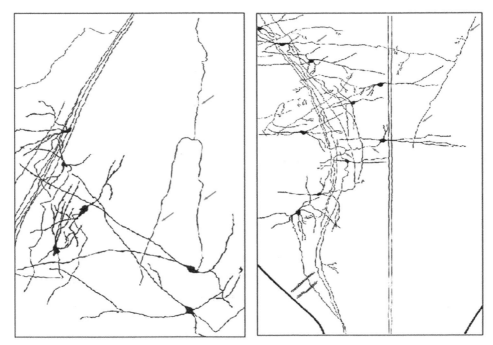

Figure 2.2 Large neurons in Nucleus GigantoCellularis (NGC) of the medullary reticular formation. All these NGC neurons have widespread dendritic arbors and long ascending or descending axonal projections. A small percentage have both ascending and descending projections (bifurcating axons marked with arrows) (Valverde, 1961, 1962). NGCs function in a vertically integrated system

electrical activity. We theorized that the important neurons for increasing generalized CNS arousal are glutamatergic, and so we arranged for the selective expression of the excitatory optogenetic protein in glutamatergic neurons. These NGC neurons, while largely quiescent during deep anesthesia, responded to optogenetic stimulation with high frequencies of firing at the same time as significant desynchronization of the cortical EEG, that is, an increase in the power of high-frequency oscillations.

We followed up the optogenetic experiments by using pharmacologic disinhibition of NGC neurons using either GABAa-antagonist bicuculline or a more specific antagonist, gabazine. Both manipulations caused a pronounced increase in neuronal firing in NGC as well as behavioral, cortical and autonomic arousal: vigorous and organized movements, increases in high frequency oscillations in the cortical EEG, and increases in respiratory frequency.

We think that these large glutamatergic neurons are kept under inhibitory control by local GABAergic neurons nearby. We predicted that optogenetically inhibiting these GABAergic neurons, which as expected are active in deep anesthesia, would release the large non-GABAergic neurons and heighten their activity and, secondly, would result in cortical arousal. These predictions were confirmed by the data.

Theory. Our theory about the central role of large medullary reticular neurons has been supported by classical neurophysiological studies and by current optogenetic studies. A series of three classical neurophysiological papers by Drew and Rossignol at the University of Montreal (1986; 1990a, b) used electrophysiological recoding of single neurons and microstimulation of the medial medullary reticular formation. Not only were discharge rates of these neurons correlated with movement but also microstimulation activated a wide variety of muscular responses. NGC neurons are leaders in the initiation of behavior. Previous studies (Brink and Pfaff, 1981; Cohen et al., 1987) had shown that medullary reticulospinal actions foster increased behavioral reactivity in the following way: electrical stimulation of hindbrain reticular formation neurons potentiate motoneuronal responses to a given strength of segmental stimulus input. That is, descending signals from the medullary reticular formation effectively increase the slope of the stimulus–response curve. Likewise, Beretzner and Brownstone (2013) inferred that activation of Lhx3/Chx10 (glutamatergic) neurons in NGC is essential for the initiation of movement. Heightened activity in NGC cells is associated with movement (Martin et al., 2010). Our theory is further supported by data in a recent paper by Capelli et al. (2017). Using optogenetics either to activate or to inhibit large glutamatergic or glycinergic neurons in the mouse medullary reticular formation, those authors achieved the theoretically predicted changes in locomotion.

Overall, it is clear that either direct activation or disinhibition of a subset of large neurons within a well-circumscribed area of the hindbrain (the medial medullary reticular formation) elicits cortical, autonomic, and motor arousal. Electrical discharges from large glutamatergic NGC neurons are likely kept under inhibitory control by smaller nearby GABA neurons. This is exactly what control system engineers would expect: the most powerful and crucial neurons should be silent when there is nothing important to signal.

Effects of Decreased Activity in NGC

In Eugene Martin's chronic electrophysiological recording experiments (Martin et al., 2010), during which he recorded the electrical activity of individual NGC neurons for a long time when the animal was awake and moving around, the *absence* of NGC neuronal discharge was associated with the animal's standing still and not doing anything. Then, action potentials would precede the initiation of locomotion. In neurophysiologist Paola Calderon's optogenetic experiments (2018), glutamatergic NGC neurons fired at very low frequencies during deep anesthesia or hypoglycemic coma. In turn, exposing these neurons to an inhibitory GABA receptor agonist, muscimol, or microinjecting an anesthetic in a manner restricted to NGC, slowed electrical activity in the cerebral cortex.

We also studied the effects of lesioning NGC and nucleus reticularis magnocellularis (NMC) (Zemlan et al., 1983). Quite large lesions were required for significant lasting effects, which comprised abnormalities of posture and locomotion.

Inputs

Sensory. In a chronic recording study in which Eugene Martin labored to be able to record from single NGC neurons while the animal was unanesthetized, moving freely, and unrestrained (Martin et al., 2010), we set five criteria for saying that the NGC neurons qualified as having an important role in generalized CNS arousal: (i) the neurons should respond to all sensory modalities tested; (ii) these responses should habituate, that is, upon repeated presentation of the same stimulus the size of the responses should decline;

(iii) higher NGC neuronal activity should be correlated with an activated cortical EEG, meaning more high-frequency activity and less low frequency; (iv) higher NGC neuronal activity should also be correlated with greater electromyogram (EMG) activity, muscular electrical discharges; and (v) NGC neuronal discharges should be associated with the initiation of movement. *All five criteria were satisfied* by the data, leading us to infer that NGC neurons are important for CNS arousal, for GA.

In these experiments, we observed excitatory responses of individual NGC neurons to all modalities tested: tactile, visual, auditory, vestibular, and olfactory. Excitation was directly linked to increase in neck muscle EMG amplitude and corresponded with increase in the power of fast oscillations (30–80 Hz) of cortical activity (EEG) and decrease in the power of slow oscillations (2–8 Hz). Because these reticular formation neurons can respond to broad ranges of stimuli with increased firing rates associated with the initiation of behavioral responses, we infer that they are part of an elementary "first responder" CNS arousal mechanism.

Synaptic. In terms of the morphology of NGC neurons, the structure of their dendritic trees provides the first clue that a primary role for these neurons is to collect information from a wide variety of sources. In 1966, Ramon-Moliner and Nauta defined the "isodendritic" dendritic tree structure as one in which the second dendritic segment is longer than the first, the third longer than the second. This dendritic design, typical of NGC, leads to a very wide dendritic spread, designed to fan out and pick up a wide variety of signals. ("Allodendritic" is exactly the opposite.)

In addition to local inputs, sources of information coming to NGC neurons have been charted by classical neuroanatomical techniques. Gallager and Pert (1978) used a "retrograde" neuroanatomical technique, in which a substance like horseradish peroxidase is placed among NGC neurons and then travels backwards up axons in order to reveal the cell bodies of origin of those axons. They charted the short-axon local connections, and they documented extensive long-axon inputs ascending from the spinal cord. Descending inputs came from the vestibular nuclei and, in the midbrain, from the midbrain reticular formation, the periaqueductal grey, the dorsal tegmentum, and the deep layers of the superior and inferior colliculi. Inputs from the nucleus of the tractus solitarius suggest signals from an autonomic system.

Other authors following Gallager and Pert have documented inputs to NGC from the periaqueductal gray of the midbrain (Fardin et al., 1984; Cottingham et al., 1987), the midbrain reticular formation (Perkins et al., 2014), the thalamus and hypothalamus (Jones and Beaudet, 1987), the cerebellum (Bharos et al., 1981; Elisevich et al., 1985), the cerebral cortex (Keiser and Kuypers, 1984; Fregosi et al., 2017), and extensive inputs ascending from the spinal cord (Peschanski and Besson, 1984).

The principle illustrated by all of these neuroanatomical results is that the networks feeding information to NGC neurons are "scaled" from the shortest to the longest. That seems to be an important feature of the vertically integrated anterior/posterior, longitudinal (A/P, L) system that produces an aroused brain. These NGC neurons are first-responders, well-connected to initiate responses to alarming stimuli.

Outputs

NGC neurons send out long axons with synapses in all the embryologically defined divisions of the nervous system (Jones and Yang, 1985; Vertes et al., 1986; Jones, 2003). In addition to local connections, they project to the pons (e.g. the pontine reticular formation) the vestibular nuclei, and, importantly for arousal stimulation, the locus coeruleus (Cedarbaum and Aghajanian, 1978). They also project to sites in the midbrain, including the midbrain reticular formation, the periaqueductal (central) gray, and the deep layers of the superior colliculus; also, projections to cerebellum.

Low road; high road. Crucially, as we ascend to reach the diencephalon, NGC outputs divide into a "low road" and "high road." Axons following the low road sweep through the medial forebrain bundle, encountering not only the dendritic fields of hypothalamic neurons (including hypocretin neurons) but even the basal forebrain where they encounter large cholinergic neurons. These cholinergic neurons have widespread effects in the cortex. I theorize that these low-road projections from NGC neurons are particularly important for supporting arousal in lower animals such as laboratory mice and rats. Their primary functions are not to regulate individual, specific behaviors, instead to change CNS state, facilitating high levels of cortical activity.

NGC axons following the high road reach the central thalamus. This is important because stimulation of the central thalamus can heighten awareness in a high-level vegetative state patient (Schiff et al., 2007) and can increase motor activity in experimental animals (Quinkert et al., 2010, 2012; Tabansky et al., 2014; Keenan et al., 2015). I theorize that these high-road functions of NGC projections are particularly important in primates, including humans (Baker et al., 2016; Schiff et al., 2007; Schiff, 2016), and *support attention and directed motor acts* through a forebrain "mesocircuit" (Schiff, 2010, 2016). According to this hypothesis, signals from central thalamus strongly drive activity in many areas of the cerebral cortex. Frontal cortical neurons in turn excite activity in a subcortical motor control region, the striatum, which in turn maintains activity in central thalamus through a two-step disinhibitory mechanism.

NGC neurons send descending axons to all levels of the spinal cord, reticulospinal neuronal axons that even reach the sacral cord, at the bottom of the neuraxis. In the words of neurophysiologist Peterson et al., (1979), stimulation of an NGC neuron will cause "monosynaptic excitation of ipsilateral motoneurons supplying axial muscles and flexor and extensor muscles in both proximal and distal parts of the limbs." Documented by Valverde (1961, 1962), some NGC neurons have bifurcating axons that contribute to both the ascending and the descending projections.

"Bowties," "fan in, fan out." As documented above, NGC neurons, studied morphologically and electrophysiologically, receive a very wide range of inputs. They also exert widespread influence throughout the CNS because of their large axonal distribution. These facts tend to support the claims of control system engineers Marie Csete and John Doyle (2004, 2005) that such fan-in/fan-out structures constitute optimal control center integrators. Such claims remain to be tested thoroughly and directly.

Functional concepts of how NGC neurons do their job tend to vary. One comparison would be between "lumpers" and "splitters." As a "lumper" I have tended theoretically to treat NGC neurons as major amplifiers, alerting the entire CNS to the need to respond to novel or dangerous stimuli. However, as a medical doctor Harvard's Veronique VanderHorst (Broom et al., 2017) "splits". She is interested in how particular functions of individual NGC neurons contribute to normal gait and, thus, how deviations from those individual specific functions could lead to neuromuscular disorders.

Bilaterality. NGC inputs and outputs are not specific to one side of the brain. In some cases individual neurons have inputs from, or outputs to, both left and right sides. Our current computational modeling effort (Bubnys et al., in press) explores the implications of descending NGC signals for the regulation of a spinal central pattern generator of locomotion.

Network theory. Some networks are far from random. The distribution of numbers of connections per node in a scale-free net can be described by a simple exponential equation; they feature a small number of nodes with tremendous numbers of connections, and many nodes with small numbers. In Barabasi's words (2003, 2009, 2011) such networks "have a power law tail." More about this is explained in Chapter 10.

This scale-free idea appears here because NGC neurons, with their profusion of both local synapses and extremely long distance projections, could typify nodes with tremendous numbers of connections. If this number of connections is indeed the case, then I am encouraged to ask whether such a hierarchical network property helps to produce the scale-free arousal behavior reported by Proekt et al (2012) and summarized in Chapter 1. Further, Barabasi (2002) thinks that such scale-free networks enjoy the property of greater error tolerance, if there are multiple hubs, an important property for regulation of generalized CNS arousal.

Genes Expressed by NGC Neurons

Do the genes expressed by NGC neurons clearly serve their functions as first-responders? The answer is a resounding yes. We have addressed the question using three approaches. First, with real-time reverse transcriptase PCR (RT-PCR) analyses of single-neuron mRNA expression in the mouse. My lab has shown that receptors consistent with participation in generalized CNS arousal are expressed by single NGC neurons. These include genes encoding receptors for the important arousal-raising peptides hypocretins, as well as genes coding for opioid peptide receptors which would decrease arousal (Martin et al., 2011). Second, genes coding for potassium ion channels Kv2.1 and Kv2.2, which allow neuronal firing at a high rate, express mRNAs in NGC. These channels are shown electrophysiologically to operate in NGC neurons as studied by patch clamp recording (Kow et al., unpublished data).

Thirdly, Inna Tabansky et al. (2018) in my lab used a new technique called retroTRAP not only to discover the full transcriptome of NGC neurons but also to list those mRNAs which are expressed selectively in NGC neurons that project to the thalamus. Those thalamic projections are important because electrical stimulation there can activate behaviors in mice (Quinkert and Pfaff, 2012; Tabansky et al., 2014) and in a human patient (Schiff et al., 2007). The transcriptome of these NGC neurons featured several patterns consistent with their known morphology and physiology: gene products that support large dendritic arbors and long axonal projections, receptors for arousal-related transmitters, and a pattern of mitochondrial gene expression that could explain the ability of these neurons to fire during the reduction or absence of oxygen (Zhou et al., 2009). Tabansky et al., (2018) also discovered an mRNA uniquely expressed in these NGC neurons with axons projecting to thalamus: endothelial nitric oxide synthase (eNOS). This discovery accompanied three other independent lines of evidence that these crucial neurons can control their own blood supply.

Origins of Origins

If activity in NGC neurons locates the origins of arousal, what are the "origins of the origins"? This chapter considers that question in three different ways.

Evolutionary origin. What about the evolutionary origins of NGC neurons? I have argued (Pfaff et al., 2012) that these NGC neurons may have evolved from the Mauthner cells in the medulla of teleost fish. Mauthner cells – with just one huge neuron per side – receive multisensory information, like NGC neurons, and by virtue of their reticulospinal axons execute escape responses from startling stimuli (Faber et al., 1989; Korn and Faber, 2005). The formation of circuits dominated by the large Mauthner cells has been described (Fetcho and McLean, 2010; Koyama et al., 2011). I propose that Mauthner cell structure and function sets up the *bauplan*, the fundamental structural plan for the GA mechanisms discussed in this book. Mauthner cells clearly are "first responders," and probably evolutionary predecessors of NGC neurons. Studies with intermediary forms, perhaps amphibia or reptiles, will add to the argument.

Embryonic origin. When my lab entered this field of work, the only evidence available indicated that in birds, large medullary reticular neurons were born both on the alar (upper) and basal plates of the embryonic brainstem (Tan and Le Douarin, 1991). We find the same result in mice, for neurons born on embryonic day 10.

Electrophysiological and behavioral origins. After mice are born, what is the origin and course of development of behavioral arousal? Preliminary evidence indicated that we should focus on the time period postnatal day 3 (P3) to postnatal day 6 (P6). So during that time period we patch clamped NGC neurons and recorded several quantitative measures (Liu et al., 2016). The following six electrophysiological characteristics increased in an orderly, statistically significant, monotonic manner over the course of P3 to P6: (i) proportion of neurons capable of firing action potential (AP) trains, dependent on the so-called "delayed rectifier" potassium currents (genes Kv2.1 and Kv2.2); (ii) AP amplitudes; (iii) AP thresholds; (iv) amplitudes of inward and outward currents; (v) amplitudes of negative peak currents; and (vi) steady state currents. These developments reflect the maturation of sodium and certain potassium channels. Similarly, all measures of locomotion (latency to first movement, total locomotion duration, net locomotion distance, and total quiescence time) also increased monotonically over P3–P6. Roughly speaking, on day P3 the pups are asleep almost all the time, while on day P6 they have a robust ability to move around. Most importantly, electrophysiological and behavioral measures mentioned above were significantly correlated. We think that the developmental increase in NGC neuronal ability to fire high-frequency trains of action potentials participates in causing the origin of behavioral responsivity during the postnatal period from P3 to P6 (Figure 2.3).

While I have emphasized the importance of NGC neurons for GA, they are not the only ones in the mammalian medulla to exert bodily state changes connected with arousal. Guyenet (1996) has reviewed roles for neurons in the ventrolateral medulla in the regulation of the autonomic nervous system. For example, the rostral ventrolateral medulla is crucial for maintaining the sympathetic autonomic control over vasomotor tone. Also, what Guyenet calls "supramedullary" structures are involved in the (parasympathetic) vagus nerve's control of cardiovascular functions.

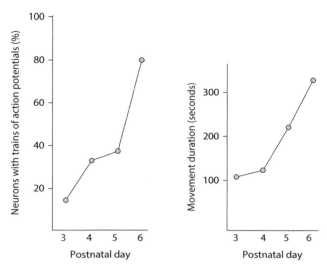

Figure 2.3 Sketch of data from Liu et al. (2016) that show a correlation between the onset of behavioral arousal in newborn mice and the development of high excitability in Nucleus GigantoCellularis (NGC) neurons in the medullary reticular formation. From postnatal day 3–6 there is a monotonic increase in the ability of NGC neurons to fire trains of spikes upon stimulation (left), which we think permits the mouse pups to develop from mainly sleeping (right, day 3) to significantly greater amounts of movement (day 6).

The raphe neurons along the midline of the medulla play important roles in responses to pain, but they are also involved in cardiovascular modulation, thermoregulation, and sexual reflexes (reviewed, Mason and Leung, 1996).

Networks

Chapter 10 elaborates on research that lends itself to "reverse engineering" the A/P, L GA system (see Figure 6.1). To do this, I invoke network theory to add insight concerning how GA works. I have emphasized that, considering the largest reticular formation neurons – certainly including NGC – with tremendously large numbers of connections, and likewise considering the excess of small neurons with only local connections, we might be dealing with a scale-free GA system (Barabasi, 2009; and for electrophysiological data, see He, 2014). Kaiser (2011) examined the question of whether human neuronal circuits are really scale-free and said "yes" for circuits in the cortex and hippocampus, albeit with different exponents in the appropriate exponential equation.

For sure, this type of system uses the largest reticular formation neurons, notably NGC, to send identical messages to a wide range of neuronal targets stretching from the lowest spinal cord to the thalamus and basal forebrain. *That is what integration means, taking many disparate signals and states and molding them to a singular initiative.*

Certainly, in such a network, NGC neurons comprise what network theorists call a "hub" or "node" (Figure 6.1). As mentioned, control system engineer, Cal Tech professor John Doyle, calls the fan-in fan-out system typified by NGC neurons a "bowtie" network which he considers ideal (Doyle and Csete, 2004, 2005).

What potentially are the other functional implications of the GA system comprising a scale-free network, if indeed that is the case? Chapter 10 addresses the issue of criticality. The main point in this chapter is that the NGC neurons can play a central role in GA networks.

Major Unanswered Questions

a. In the retroTRAP experiment (Tabansky et al., 2018) we discovered a large number of messenger RNAs that were significantly enriched in NGC neurons with ascending axons. What are all those gene products doing? Is there a corresponding set expressed in NGC neurons with descending axons?

b. While I have emphasized the powerful amplification of GA signaling by NGC neurons, others, such as neurologist Veronique vanderHorst at Harvard, are interested in the particularity of how individual sub-classes of NGC neurons contribute to normal gait. What are the trade-offs between the powerful but undifferentiated GA signaling, compared to the particularity required for coordinated movement?

c. It is easy to think about large glutamatergic NGC neurons surrounded by inhibitory glycinergic or GABAergic neurons which keep the firing rates of the large neurons in check. But is that really true? The Calderon et al.'s (2018) report seems to indicate that it is true. But, in general, what are the relationships between the giant NGC neurons and other cells nearby. How do these neuronal groups articulate with each other?

d. Some NGC neurons are connected through gap junctions, allowing for a rapid spread of excitation among them. Does that mean they are well suited to act as "first responders"?

e. Tabansky's (2018) four converging lines of evidence suggest that some NGC neurons can regulate their own blood supply. What are the functional consequences of those data?

f. We have small bits of evidence that small numbers of NGC neurons lie outside the blood–brain barrier. What substances in the blood would influence the activities of these neurons, and how might these influence the behavior?

Behavioral evidence cited in Chapter 1 suggests that GA mechanisms near the phase transition between inactivity and arousal have a "scaling property" – self-similarity of dynamics over a very wide range of magnitudes – that yield data following a power law. Does this scaling property originate with NGC neurons? I note that such scaling is not confined to the nervous system and behavior. For example, Peter Reich at the University of Minnesota has reported "universal scaling" of respiration, metabolism, and size in plants (Reich et al., 2006).

Summary

Two features of NGC neurons enable them to function as "master cells" for generalized CNS arousal. First, they feature a tremendous range of lengths of axonal projections from local connections, through medium length, through very long. This range supports the creation of a vertically integrated anterior/posterior longitudinal system. Second, they respond to a very wide distribution of inputs, and distribute their responses widely. By means of their fan-in/fan-out property, they fulfill two of the operating requirements for a generalized arousal system: marked convergence of inputs and divergence of outputs. Further, Tabansky's (2018) discovery of a unique relation between these neurons and their blood supply suggests that NGC cells could respond to humoral signals as well. All of these properties indicate that they can perform their function as "first responders," initiating fast responses to alarming and other salient stimuli.

Since these neurons represent the origins of arousal, the physical location where arousal originates, it was possible, in this chapter, to put forward the "origins of the origins of arousal" (i) in evolutionary terms; and (ii) during early brain development; and (iii) first awakenings just after birth.

Finally, the high channel capacity, the signaling power of NGC neuron strengthens the notion that major themes from the neuroscience literature cited in this book are actually related to each other. The A/P, L ladder-like signaling makes for high connectivity of GA systems and for the essence of "integration" by virtue of sending the same message to many different outlets. If this GA net is really scale-free, then certain scale-free features of GA-related behavior might be predicted. Further, I conjecture that the basic elements of GA systems are present universally in vertebrate brains – NGC neurons can be thought of as descendants of fish brain Mauthner nerve cells.

Pons

Chapter 3

Many excellent neuroscientists have worked on the neuroanatomy, neurophysiology, and functions of specific cell groups in the pons (recall Figure 2.1). This chapter explores how their collective actions can be conceived as contributing to generalized arousal (GA). My focus is on whether and how their contributions fit into the theoretical approach to GA presented in Chapter 1.

Reviewing the classical literature on this embryologically defined segment ("metencephalon") of the lower brainstem, as well as the current literature through 2017, I can propose at least three ways in which nerve cell groups in the pons contribute importantly to GA. First, involvement of the locus coeruleus (LC) with neuroendocrinology and other aspects of hypothalamic function seems unmistakable. Second, controls of the viscera – internal organs of the body, mainly located in the great cavities of the trunk, e.g., heart and the cardiovascular system, lungs, intestines – come into play with respect to neurons in the pons, especially the control of breathing, obviously connected with arousal and emotion. Third, large neurons in the pontine reticular formation play important roles which affect the stages of sleep.

Locus Coeruleus

Named originally by human gross anatomists who were struck by the cerulean blue color of a cadaver's blood supply there, this tightly packed group of neurons in the posterior pons, LC, plays a major role in regulating brain arousal. Following a small group of brilliant Swedish histochemists, Larry Swanson, then at Washington University of Saint Louis (Swanson and Hartman, 1974), used fluorescent antibodies against the enzyme that converts dopamine into the neurotransmitter noradrenaline (also called norepinephrine) in order to describe LC, the largest and most distinctive collection of noradrenergic cell bodies that yield the wide-ranging fiber system which supplies noradrenaline to the entire forebrain.

Craig Berridge (2008; Berridge and Waterhouse, 2003) emphasized the impressive wake-promoting actions of the LC projections to the preoptic area and the medial septum of the forebrain, and discerned which adrenergic subtypes are responsible for these actions. The subsequent effects on the electrical activity of the ancient forebrain limbic system and cerebral cortex are strong and reliable. For example, increasing the electrical activity of neurons in LC by the local application of a cholinergic drug caused activation of the cortical electroencephalogram, changing the recordings from low-frequency high-amplitude to high-frequency low-amplitude waves (Berridge and Foote, 1991). It also caused intense theta rhythms (6–7 waves per second) in the hippocampus, a sign of activation.

Putting this work into the context of sleep–wake daily cycles and circadian rhythms, Gary Aston-Jones et al. (2001), now chief of neuroscience at Rutgers University, used a form of neuroanatomical tracing that is not limited to one axon–synaptic connection but can reveal an entire series of connections. With this, he traced connections between the central "biological clock" of the brain, the suprachiasmatic nucleus of the hypothalamus, to the LC. These connections, importantly through waystations called the paraventricular and dorsomedial nuclei of the hypothalamus, explain how the daily light rhythm can affect the arousing properties of LC activity.

Subsequently, Aston-Jones and Cohen (2005) pointed out that in primates like monkeys, LC neurons have two different rhythms of electrical activity: "tonic," i.e., activity when not engaged in a particular task, and "phasic" meaning activity "driven by the outcome of task-related decision processes." Tonic implies a fairly constant frequency of firing for a long time, which is higher if the animal is attentive and alert. Phasic implies higher levels of activity driven by the occurrence of a goal-relevant stimulus. The novel idea of their theory is that frontal cortical neurons can actually modulate temporal patterns of LC activity during task performance, optimizing the dynamic properties of attention-dependent behavioral circuits (pp. 418–20).

To broaden coverage from Aston-Jones' and Cohen's comprehensive reviews, we envision how daily arousal rhythms depend on the outputs from the suprachiasmatic nucleus (SCN) of the hypothalamus. The links from the SCN use at least three pathways. Through these multiple connections, there are links to orexinergic systems, LC, and to the reticular formation:

i.   There is a diffusible signal from SCN to neural sites regulating locomotor activity (Silver et al., 1996). The precise targets of this diffusible signal remain to be identified, but easily could include LC.

ii. There is a very extensive set of multisynaptic connections from SCN to numerous brain regions (Morin, 2013).

iii. Indirect routes, where the SCN modulation of hormonal and feeding rhythms influences many hormones that act systemically – at many neural and peripheral loci (Pfaff et al., 2018, principles #16, 17) – to affect activity levels; e.g., ghrelin (LeSauter et al., 2009).

With all of this classical work heightening our interest in LC, is there a new and correct summary of what "job" it has in the biologically adaptive regulation of GA? A reasonable place to begin answering that question is to note its inputs. What signals are LC neurons listening to?

Three ideas stand out as answers to this question. First, hypothalamic inputs to LC are strong, with an emphasis on hypocretin/orexin. Second, both peptide and steroid hormones influence LC neurons. Third, afferents from visceral neurons are prominent.

I will review the literature with those ideas in mind, but without being limited by them. For example, Cedarbaum and Aghajanian (1978) used a classical neuroanatomical retrograde tracing technique to show large numbers of neurons projecting to LC from the forebrain and hypothalamus, namely the insular cortex; the central nucleus of the amygdala; the medial, lateral, and magnocellular preoptic areas; the bed nucleus of the stria terminalis; and the dorsomedial, paraventricular, and lateral hypothalamic areas. Their results have been repeated many times by studies showing impressive inputs from limbic structures such as the central nucleus of the amygdala and inputs from the hypothalamus and preoptic area. Cedarbaum and Aghajanian also reported retrogradely labeled neurons in the reticular formation, the midbrain central gray, and from a visceral-receiving zone, and concluded that the LC must play a role in behavioral arousal mechanisms and autonomic regulation. Garcia-Rill et al. (1983) and the Kiehn lab (Caggiano et al., 2017) discovered inputs from the region of the midbrain from which locomotion can be initiated and locomotor speed controlled. In a smaller study, Michel Jouvet's lab in Lyon, France (Sakai et al., 1976), produced similar data showing some afferent projections to the LC complex from visceral signaling centers such as the nucleus of the solitary tract, the dorsal motor nucleus of the vagus, and from hypothalamic and preoptic areas.

Rita Valentino and Elizabeth Van Bockstaele (Reyes et al., 2005) concentrated on the ultrastructural features of hypothalamic afferents to the LC. The hypothalamic paraventricular nucleus set axons that synapsed on noradrenergic neurons in LC. Retrograde transport from the LC combined with immunocytochemical detection of hypothalamic neuropeptides showed that some of the projecting neurons express the stress-related corticotrophic releasing factor (CRF).

How is it possible to keep LC activity under control? One means is the inhibitory transmitter GABA. In the dendritic field of LC, a large percentage of small cells stained for GABA (Aston-Jones et al., 2004). Ultrastructural analyses revealed synaptic contacts between these GABA neurons and LC neurons. Another means of direct relevance to medicine and public health would be opioid peptides.

Rita Valentino and her colleagues (Kreibich et al., 2008), referring to the fact that both mu and kappa opioid receptors are expressed in or near LC, performed an experiment in which a chemical compound that is active through kappa opioid receptors was microinfused into LC. The drug did not alter spontaneous discharges of LC neurons but attenuated responses to various stimuli. Importantly, activating kappa opioid receptors also reduced neuronal response hypotensive stress, an effect mediated by corticotrophic releasing factor (CRF, see below), thus eliciting a theme which will be discussed again: the roles of CRF and LC neurons in processing stressful events and environments.

Hypothalamic hypocretin/orexin inputs. Perhaps the newest and biggest story about arousal-related inputs to LC involves the hypothalamic peptide that was cloned by Luis de Lecea ("hypocretin") and also by Masami Yanagasawa ("orexin"). As summarized by Craig Berridge's lab (España et al., 2005), hypocretin/orexin neurons give rise to an extensive projection system, including the LC. Hypocretin neurons projecting to the LC were located primarily within the dorsal half of the hypocretin cell group. Robert Moore and his colleagues (2001) extended work in this field to the human brain, and confirmed hypocretin projections to LC as part of a wide distribution of axons. Thus, we can argue for LC neurons as crucial for CNS arousal in the human brain as well as laboratory animals.

Matthew Carter and Luis de Lecea (2009a) showed that optogenetic stimulation of Hcrt neurons was sufficient to increase the probability of an awakening event during both slow-wave and rapid eye movement (REM) sleep, and subsequently wanted to know whether Hcrt-mediated sleep-to-wake transitions are affected by the phase of the light–dark daily cycle and sleep pressure. In their words, "stimulation of Hcrt neurons increased the probability of an awakening event throughout the entire light/dark period but that this effect was diminished with 'sleep pressure' induced by 2 or 4 h of sleep deprivation." Knowing that activity in LC neurons correlates with behavioral arousal, Carter et al. (2010) used optogenetic tools delivered in viral vectors to demonstrate a "frequency-dependent, causal relationship among LC firing, cortical activity, sleep-to-wake transitions and general locomotor arousal." Further analyses (Carter et al., 2012) showed that inhibiting locus neurons during unilateral hypocretin stimulation reduced sleep-to-wake transitions, whereas optogenetic stimulation of LC neurons facilitated hypocretin effects on waking. Overall, Carter et al., (2013) concluded that "noradrenergic neurons in LC are particularly important for mediating the effects of hypocretin neurons on arousal."

Hormonal inputs. Until now, all the inputs to LC that I have considered have been neuronal. But what about hormonal? It turns out that two classes of hormones, steroids and peptide hormones, should be addressed. The simpler example features the steroid hormone estradiol. The laboratory of Esther Sabban (Serova et al., 2002) studied effects of estradiol administration on gene expression in LC. It might be possible to say that the most uniquely important gene in these neurons expresses the mRNA for the enzyme tyrosine hydroxylase, the rate-limiting enzyme for making norepinephrine. The estrogen effect was as great as threefold over control. The gene for another enzyme involved in norepinephrine synthesis, dopamine beta-hydroxylase (DBH), had its mRNA levels similarly increased. Analyses of the molecular mechanisms were straightforward: estrogens were acting through these genes' promoters in a manner that required estrogen receptor alpha. Thinking that estrogenic hormones are likely involved in the gender-specific differences in coping with stress, Sabban and her colleagues (Serova et al., 2005) studied their effects on the kinds of gene expression and physiological responses to immobilization stress. In several respects, estrogen administration reversed the effects of immobilization stress. For example, the elevation of DBH mRNA in LC was reversed, as well as the effect of stress on blood pressure.

The hypothalamic neuroendocrine peptide corticotrophic releasing hormone (CRH) in LC is a huge story. Rita Valentino and Gary Aston-Jones (see Valentino et al 1983) used immunohistochemical techniques to characterize CRH, aka corticotropin-releasing factor (CRF), innervation of LC. CRF-immunoreactive fibers were identified in the LC. Subsequent studies localizing both CRF and tyrosine hydroxylase (for making norepinephrine) showed CRF-immunoreactive fibers overlapping with tyrosine hydroxylase-staining processes of LC neurons. The same team found that CRF administered intraventricularly increased the discharge rates of LC neurons (Valentino et al., 1983). A similar effect on electrical firing rate was observed during direct application of CRF to LC neurons by pressure microapplication. Later, Prouty et al. (2017) analyzed that these increases in electrical activity are dependent on CRF receptor subtype 1. The excitatory pathway uses cyclic AMP (cAMP) intracellular signaling cascades resulting in changes in certain potassium conductances. The results of the new work were tricky. Whether the CRF would increase or decrease activity depended on the exact dose used. The authors inferred that stress may differentially affect ongoing excitatory synaptic transmission in LC depending on exactly how much CRF is released from presynaptic terminals.

Further light was shed on the excitatory effects of CRF by Rita Valentino and Elizabeth Van Bockstaele (see Valentino et al 2001). They identified separate excitatory (glutamate) and inhibitory (GABA) amino acid afferents to LC. Most important, many synaptic terminals that contained immunolabeling for both CRF and glutamate were observed, but relatively few terminals exhibited immunolabeling for both GABA and CRF. To my mind this co-localization of CRF with the excitatory amino acid glutamate supports the discoveries of increases in LC activity due to CRF. Valentino and Foote (1988) extended their previous work to test the hypothesis that CRF is released from axons innervating the noradrenergic neurons of the LC and serves to activate these neurons during stress responses.

Specifically, the effects of exogenous CRH on the electrophysiological activity of LC neurons in unanesthetized rats were characterized: intracerebroventricular CRH caused a dose-dependent increase in locus neurons' spontaneous discharge rates. The effects of CRH administration on sensory-evoked activity of LC neurons were also determined, and here the CRF effect was not nearly as impressive as the effect on tonic activity.

Visceral inputs. Strong inputs to LC comes from cardiovascular and vagal afferents. With electrophysiological techniques, Elam et al. (1984) studied the effects of activation of blood–volume receptors or arterial baroreceptors on the firing rate of single cells in LC, which turned out to be more sensitive to blood–volume expansion than peripheral autonomic nerves. Blood pressure elevation caused an immediate reduction in both the firing rate of LC cells. These authors followed up that study (Elam et al., 1985) with the reverse manipulation by showing that activity in LC was increased during blood–volume depletion.

Finally, Elam et al. used electrophysiological techniques to show that distension of the urinary bladder, the distal colon, rectum, or the stomach causes pronounced activation responses of locus neurons (Elam et al., 1986). In their words, their "results implicate the locus coeruleus as a pivotal system by which autonomic or visceral functions can affect behavior and, conversely, by which environmental stress can affect autonomic functions."

Some of the elctrophysiological actions of inputs to LC are complex. Takigawa and Mogenson (1977) found that, while stimulation of some autonomic nerves produced mainly excitation of LC neurons, stimulation of others (e.g., the vagus nerve) produced mainly inhibition or inhibition followed by excitation. Convergence of inputs from different sources onto individual locus neurons was common.

As noted above, the inputs to LC from the phylogenetically ancient forebrain, structures such as the amygdala and the hypothalamus, are impressive. Rita Valentino's team (Curtis et al., 2002) looked for which brain regions might be responsible for the effect of hypotensive stress to cause CRF release within the LC. Clearly, lesions of the central nucleus of the amygdala greatly reduced the stress effect on LC. To support this, a substantial number of CRF-expressing neurons in the central nucleus of the amygdala were retrogradely labeled from the LC. Their electrophysiological and anatomical findings implicated amygdala as a primary source of CRF that activates the LC during hypotensive stress.

Regarding inputs, I indicated earlier that regulation of breathing is related in an obvious manner to arousal and emotion. Recent work (Yackle et al., 2017) demonstrates how this this might work, regarding LC. The authors used several modern neuroscience techniques to link neurons that regulate breathing rhythms to activity in the LC, arousal-regulating as covered above. Specifically, the authors identified a gene, cadherin-9 (Cdh9), most selectively expressed in a brainstem breathing control center in neurons of the preBotC, a critical region generating inspiratory rhythm. Using genetic technology, they destroyed preBotC neurons that coexpress two genes, Cdh9 and Dbx1. As a result of such ablation, mice were calmer, their arousal was decreased, and their breathing slowed but otherwise appeared normal (perhaps as in human meditation techniques). The authors propose that these effects depend on axonal projections to the LC, where, with preBotC neurons expressing those two genes ablated, immediate early gene expression (usually associated with elevated neural activity) was reduced and was less reactive to environmental changes and to physical restraint.

The implications of this work for medicine and public health are manifold. For example, since hypersecretion of CRF has been hypothesized to occur in depression, Curtis and

Valentino (1994) have considered that CRF hypersecretion in LC could be responsible for some characteristics of depression. They tested this hypothesis using electrophysiological recordings of LC neurons. Chronic (continuous) administration of two antidepressants inhibited LC activation by a hypotensive, stress, and administration of two other antidepressants altered responses to repeated sciatic nerve stimulation in a manner opposite to the effect produced by CRF. Both these results suggest that some antidepressants may oppose CRF actions in LC. Wood and Valentino (2017) have expanded our thinking about the contributions of the LC-norepinephrine system to stress-induced cardiovascular disease. They argue that "differences in coping strategy determine individual differences in social stress-induced cardiovascular vulnerability." The correlated differences in the regulation of LC neuronal activity "would translate to differences in cardiovascular regulation and may serve as the basis for individual differences in the cardiopathological consequences of social stress."

Outputs. Basically, LC axons and synapses supply the forebrain with norepinephrine (noradrenaline). Axons go to the phylogenetically ancient forebrain, the "limbic system," including the hippocampus, the septum, and the amygdala. They even go so far as the olfactory bulb. A rich supply innervates cell groups in the hypothalamus. LC axons also project to the thalamus, the midbrain, the cerebellum and the spinal cord (reviewed, Saper, 2000).

Functions. It would be easy to think of the noradrenergic outputs from LC simply as "waking up" the entire brain. However, a more sophisticated view comes from the recent theoretical paper of Trevor Robbins (Trofimova and Robbins, 2016) at the University of Cambridge. These authors talk about three neurotransmitter systems called "monoaminergic," referring to chemical amino groups (one nitrogen, three hydrogens). Consider noradrenaline (norepinephrine). They point out that these locus outputs "may act differently upon the level of arousal, type of receptors and their precise location within those neural systems controlling behavior." For example, "under conditions of hyperarousal, noradrenalin release in the prefrontal cortex impairs working memory, but enhances long term memory consolidation in the amygdala." The noradrenergic function of "attention to novelty and orientation" is always emphasized in Robbins' writing.

LC responses decline ("habituate") when sensor stimuli are presented repeatedly. The noradrenergic system is most active during the waking state (Aston-Jones et al., 2005). If indeed noradrenaline neurons in LC are especially important for their "exploration and exploitation of behavioural alternatives," then we can understand how Trevor Robbins assigns their roles for the "expansion of behavioral alternatives, especially noted under conditions of novel or unpredictable events."

When we hear about three monoaminergic neurotransmitter systems as *opposed* to generalized CNS arousal, we realize that a false dichotomy has been constructed. Really, the proper formulation of the question is not specific systems *or* a deeper more generalized force for the initiation of behavior. Instead, the answer is the set of three (and more) specific systems *and* generalized CNS arousal. The differential equation (1.1) proposed in Chapter 1 offers a more universal solution than the simple specialized systems. Note that the constants in the differential equation can be different for different individuals, developmental stages, and environments.

Gary Aston-Jones and his colleagues (1996) put a slightly different theoretical spin on their thinking about LC function. Data gathered up to the point of their writing linked the LC both to the EEG and autonomic responses following emotionally arousing stimuli. This argument is not inconsistent with Robbins' point of view – it simply shifts the emphasis to emotionally significant stimuli and responses.

In summary, a tremendous amount of neuroanatomical and electrophysiological evidence, correlated with behavioral observations, tell us that LC neurons contribute to cognitive and emotional functions through their effects on CNS arousal (Sara and Bouret, 2012). Which of these contributions are essential and unique will be revealed by selective *reductions* of LC neuronal subtypes.

Pedunculopontine Nucleus

There are special reasons for paying close attention to neurons in the pedunculopontine (PPT) nucleus (reviewed, Garcia-Rill, 2015a, b). Both glutamatergic and cholinergic neurons in that location offer excitatory inputs to the central thalamus. Pay attention to that connection because electrical stimulation can activate behaviors in normal and brain-damaged mice (Quinkert et al., 2010, 2012; Tabansky et al., 2014) and can have amazing therapeutic effects in a high-end vegetative state patient (Schiff et al., 2007). Deep-brain stimulation, so long a tool for neurologists treating patients with Parkinson's disease, is now being considered by neurologists for application to the PPT nucleus as well. Benarroch (2013), aware that these PPT neurons are involved in mechanisms of cortical arousal, envisions the development of deep-brain stimulation there for several kinds of patients. Garcia-Rill et al. (2015), likewise, see the role of PPT neurons in arousal, and also a role for deep-brain stimulation of those neurons in treating movement disorders. Roles for PPT neurons in arousal recently have been reviewed (Mena-Segovia and Bolam, 2017).

Intellectually, the most interesting development regarding these neurons has to do with our management of sleep states, in the words of Clif Saper, Chief of Neurology at Harvard Medical School, "the ability to fall asleep or to snap out of sleep into wakefulness." For what Saper et al. (2010) calls "the sleep/wake switch," cholinergic neurons in the PPT nucleus, i.e., cells that project to the central thalamus, are crucial.

Further, Saper has been thinking about a different "switch" in the sleep system, one that manages the transitions between REM sleep, associated with dreaming, and other sleep states (Fuller et al., 2007). Here is the key idea: give a neuroscientist a set of neurons "X" that inhibits firing in a different set of neurons "Y," under conditions where Y neurons also inhibit X (with a time delay), and you have created a situation that leads to bistable states, flipping one way or the other as a function of time. Lu et al (2006) have detected just that, in the upper pons and lower midbrain with one such cell group (call it X) being GABAergic neurons in the ventrolateral periqueductal gray (central gray) and the other (call it Y) being the formerly obscure sublateralodorsal nucleus. Thus, a frequent theme in coming years for the neuroscience of sleep will be the physiology and molecular biology of mutually inhibitory neuronal groups.

A side point: part of the GA arousing properties of the PPT nucleus may derive from its close relations with the Parabrachial region (Fuller et al., 2011). This possibility remains to be worked out (see below).

Pontine Reticular Formation

Neurons in at least two locations of the pontine reticular formation regulate different aspects of sleep. On the one hand, Ito et al (2002) used intracellular recordings of pontine reticular formation neurons before and during the onset of the REM phase of sleep to demonstrate sustained membrane depolarization (activation) in REM sleep as compared with more polarized membrane potential levels in slow-wave sleep. Van Someren and Cluydts (2017) review the literature and highlight large cholinergic neurons in the medial pontine reticular formation (p. 2297). Also, Brown and McCarley (2006) used pharmacological, lesion, and single-unit recording techniques to identify a region of the pontine reticular formation just ventral to the LC as critically involved in the generation of REM sleep.

Everything about the concepts of the physiology of these pontine neurons should be viewed in light of the early work of the Scheibels using the Golgi stain, a silver stain that permits the neuroscientist to see the entire neuron: the cell body, the dendritic tree, and the axonal distribution. Once again, these connectivities seem "scale-free": large numbers of local connections and certain synapses which are very far away from the cell bodies. The conclusions of the Scheibels (see Jasper, 1958) about the organization of the brainstem's reticular core were based on observations of more than 4000 brains in species ranging from mice and rats to monkeys and human infants. They emphasized large numbers of heterogeneous afferents upon single reticular neurons and tremendously long anterior/posterior-running axonal systems. This is a fan-in–fan-out system with wide dendritic trees that respect what they call "segmental signatures" (p. 35), which is why I have divided this book along embryologically defined A/P divisions. In addition to the long-distance signaling, large reticular neurons, in the words of the Scheibels "solicit the interest" (p. 40) of nearby reticular neurons, thus potentially causing an avalanche of electrical activity. This structure may possibly lead to a scale-free network of potential interest for the generation of scale-free behavior (Proekt et al., 2012). The Scheibels observed large reticular neurons with bifurcating axons whose major limbs projected rostrally and caudally, giving off collaterals along the way. Thus, for sleep regulation from the pons, as for NGC neurons in the medulla (Chapter 1), we are dealing with an anterior/posterior longitudinally (A/P, L) extended system.

So, on the one hand, large pontine reticular neurons could function importantly as hubs (notes) in A/P, L distributed nets, which would be important for adding stability to these nets (see Chapter 10). On the other hand, these giant neurons are understudied. They need to be recorded in unrestrained behaving animals. Their transcriptomes need to be defined (cf., for NGC, Tabansky et al., 2018). A lot of work remains to be done in the pons.

Parabrachial Nucleus

Continuing themes from above, neurons in the group called the parabrachial nucleus are concerned with visceral functions as far as arousal is concerned. Harvard professor Clif Saper's thinking (2016), emphasizing autonomic regulations, echoes his classical neuroanatomical work (Saper and Loewy, 1980). In that paper he showed very proximal projections to the serotonin-producing groups nearby the raphe nuclei projections to the thalamus and hypothalamus, but also long-ranging axons to subnuclei in the amygdala. In fact, some parabrachial neurons have axons reaching specific areas of the cerebral cortex. This pattern repeats the "scale-free network" theme that I raised in Chapter 2. The import of parabrachial nucleus outputs for neuroendocrine functions, autonomic functions, and breathing is obvious. Another way of putting this point is that arousal systems co-opt specific autonomic regulatory features in the service of CNS-wide coordination.

Breathing. More specifically, the Saper team (Kaur et al., 2013) tested possible roles for glutamatergic neurons in the parabrachial nucleus in "hypercapnic arousal." The word hypercapnia refers to abnormally elevated carbon dioxide (CO_2) levels in the blood. Such an elevation is expected to trigger a reflex which increases breathing. Deleting glutamatergic neurons in the parabrachial nucleus caused a significant delay in the ability of the brain to arouse following the onset of hypercapnia. During extensive experiments (Yokota et al., 2015), the authors found that hypercapnia activated the expression of an immediate early gene, c-Fos, expression in certain parabrachial neurons. In order to determine exactly which neurons in the parabrachial contributed to respiratory stimulation, Chamberlin and Saper (1994) used microinjections of the excitatory transmitter, glutamate. Far rostral neurons and most lateral neurons excited heavier breathing.

Other cell groups in the posterior aspects of the ventral and lateral pons also are essential for the regulation of respiratory rhythms closely connected with emotional arousal. As reviewed by Del Negro et al. (2018) inspiratory responses depend on a specific, molecularly defined subgroup of neurons in the "pre-Boetzinger complex" (named after a German Boetzinger wine shared at the scientific meeting). Required for inspiration are neurons that express the homeobox gene Dbx6: "*Dbx1*-knockout mice do not form a recognizable preBötComplex and die at birth because they do not breathe; *in vitro* preparations from these mice do not generate inspiratory rhythm." Further, neurons near the facial nucleus in the ventral and lateral pons drive active expiration. Some of these neurons are chemically sensitive and thus could respond to levels of CO_2 in the blood. The molecular signatures of these latter neurons remain to be discovered.

The Saper team also worked on outputs relevant to the cardiovascular system. Chamberlin and Saper (1992) used microstimulation to reveal pressor-tachycardic responses that mapped to the outer edge of the external lateral subnucleus while depressor-bradycardic responses were elicited from stimuli near the dorsal lateral subnucleus. In their words, "these observations indicate that the PB contains at least two distinct neuronal systems that are potently and oppositely involved in cardiovascular control." The underlying meaning of these oppositional responses remains to be worked out.

Similar themes emerge when we talk about inputs to the parabrachial nucleus. King (1980) described major inputs to the solitary complex, a visceral and gustatory receiving zone. Likewise, Hermann and Rogers (1985) used both neuroanatomical and electrophysiological methods to reveal hepatic (liver) and gustatory (taste) inputs to different regions of the solitary nucleus, both of which, in turn, project to a specific region of the parabrachial nucleus. The two types of signals, visceral and gustatory, augment each other in their ability to excite electrical activity in individual parabrachial neurons. This same group found breathing-related inputs from the medulla, in previous work. It is easy to understand that breathing and gastrointestinal functions should be relevant to arousal signaling.

Reflections

Regarding the pons, I have emphasized neuroendocrine links, regulation of the viscera, breathing, and sleep in my analyses of mechanisms underlying arousal. These specific physiological systems are effectively co-opted in the service of generalized CNS arousal. Since I have never worked in the pons (the "metencephalon"), I have relied entirely on published sources from other labs. It appears to me as though four cell groups covered in this chapter – LC, the PPT nucleus, the pontine reticular formation, and the parabrachial nucleus – contribute to and strengthen the more abstract idea I posed in Chapter 2: scale-free networks that produce high states of GA.

Match to theory. In particular, the large pontine reticular formation neurons look well-suited to provide an additional "hub" (node) in GA networks that may prove to be scale-free. If so, they match the A/P, L formulation from Chapters 1 and 2, joining therefore with NGC and providing more stability to the GA system. LC probably provides the same functions: local signaling, long-distance signaling, and steady contribution to GA.

As we march up the brainstem from the most posterior level, the embryologically defined myencephalon (medulla), to the metencephalon (pons), and then to the mes-encephalon (midbrain), we are – even in this chapter – facing a division in the road to complete scientific explanation. Neuroscientists are familiar with the division into "splitters" (emphasizing cell-to-cell differences and distinctions in morphological and functional results) *versus* "lumpers" (instead, emphasizing overriding principles and themes in a field of work). This chapter has been "lumping," passing over details to get to the main points; those points have comprised structure–function relationships because not enough molecular biology – serious studies of transcriptional regulation – has been done in the pons compared to, for example, the hypothalamus.

Regarding lumping versus splitting, my scientific description of generalized CNS arousal mechanisms subscribes (in grander words) to Philip Ball's description of the new book *Scale* by the theoretical physicist Geoffrey West. Ball's review points out the distinction between Plato's approach, which speaks of "similarities, patterns, and universals," and Aristotle's, which focuses on "differences, variations, and specifics." As we leave the pons and approach the midbrain, it is clear I have adopted the Platonic route, and can only hope that my Aristotelean neurobiological friends will stay on board.

Midbrain

Moving up the brainstem, we have traversed the embryological levels called myencephalon (medulla) and metencephalon (pons), now to reach the mesencephalon (midbrain). After covering the inputs and outputs of the midbrain periaqueductal gray (central gray), I will discuss two neurotransmitters obviously associated with CNS arousal: dopamine and serotonin. Finally, I will describe briefly a debate about outputs ascending through the midbrain and their relative importance for generalized arousal (GA) and consciousness. Some groups think that outputs to the basal forebrain are crucial, while others emphasize outputs to the central thalamus. In my opinion, both are important for GA. The "low road" to the basal forebrain in both lower animals and humans supports CNS state changes from less to more aroused. The "high road" through the central thalamus, in humans, supports consciousness and attention to sensory stimuli as well as permitting guided movements.

Periaqueductal Gray (Central Gray)

Inputs. What signals are periaqueductal gray neurons listening to? Al Beitz (1982) used a retrograde transport technique to find out. The largest cortical input to this midbrain region arises from the medial prefrontal cortex. The basal forebrain provides a significant input to the periaqueductal gray. The hypothalamus sends the largest descending input to the central gray, while the medullary and pontine reticular formation provides the largest input to the periaqueductal gray, ascending from the lower brain stem.

Results from Professor Joan Morrell, in my lab (Morrell et al., 1981), agree with that of Beitz. In our study, retrogradely labeled neurons were most numerous in the reticular formation, specifically in the pontine and medullary gigantocellular (NGC) regions and in the sensory trigeminal complex. This result with NGC offers further evidence for my theoretical assertion of the ladder-like nature of anterior/posterior longitudinally (A/P, L) reticular formation signaling, featuring local medium-length and very long axons that overlap along the anterior/posterior (A/P) axis.

Likewise, Menétrey and de Pommery (1991) studied the locations of spinal cells, including autonomic signals, projecting rostrally to central areas that process viscero-ception and visceronociception. They showed that the spinomesencephalic tract reaches the periaqueductal gray and adjacent areas.

In the Department of Physiology at the University of Bristol, Thelma Lovick (2016) studied afferent input from small-caliber axons innervating the urinary bladder, i.e., visceral sensation. Some of these connections that signal bladder filling activate a spino-bulbo-spinal loop, which relays in the midbrain periaqueductal gray. These small-caliber bladder afferents are normally silent but are activated in inflammatory bladder states and by intense distending pressure, i.e., visceral pain.

The midbrain central gray also receives significant ascending signals that use GA-related transmitters originating from neurons in the medulla. In a comprehensive study, Herbert and Saper (1992) used combinations of retrograde neuroanatomical tracers, anterograde, and immunocytochemistry for enzymes that synthesize *norepinephrine* (noradrenaline) and *epinephrine* (adrenaline) for two purposes: to demonstrate adrenergic and noradrenergic fibers in the central gray, and to discover the neurons from which they ascended. The most striking findings were that neurons in the noradrenergic A1 group medulla and A2 group in the medial part of the nucleus of the solitary tract, and in the adrenergic C1 group in the rostral ventrolateral medulla and C3 group in the rostral dorsomedial medulla are the sources of noradrenergic and adrenergic fibers in the central gray. These projections certainly are sufficient to support an important role for the central gray in the regulation of GA. They support GA related to stress and autonomic drive. Further, these ascending adrenergic projections supply the most important aminergic modulator of the hypothalamic/pituitary/adrenal axis in the context of stress, which is an aspect of GA in the context of this book's data and theory.

Outputs. Jerry Eberhart, working with Professor Morrell in my lab (Eberhart et al., 1985), studied ascending projections from the midbrain periaqueductal gray using tritiated amino acid autoradiography. In addition to local projections within the midbrain, ascending fibers follow two trajectories. The *ventral* projection passes through the ventral tegmental region of Tsai and the medial forebrain bundle to reach the hypothalamus, preoptic area, basal forebrain, and even the frontal cortex. The *dorsal* periventricular projection terminates in the midline and intralaminar thalamic nuclei. Eberhart's results illustrate two important points. First, the distribution of very short, local projections combined with very long projections to basal forebrain underline the argument in Chapter 10 about scale-free distributions. Second, the dorsal high road and ventral low road trajectories will be highlighted at the end of this chapter, as they feed naturally into Chapters 5 and 6.

Regarding the concept of a low road and high road from the midbrain forward, the results of Edwards and de Olmos (1976) agree with Eberhart's conclusions. De Olmos reported that the ascending projections of the midbrain's cuneiform nucleus included more ventrally directed fibers which distribute to the posterior hypothalamus and zona incerta. The second division of fiber ascends through midline and intralaminar nuclei, completely encircling the mediodorsal nucleus. One part of Eberhart's and de Olmos' interest was addressed by the lab of James Herman at the University of Cincinnati (Myers et al., 2017). The Herman lab deals with mechanisms of responses to stress, defined as "a real or perceived threat to homeostasis or well-being." Both the endocrine and the behavioral responses to stress depend on the paraventricular hypothalamic nucleus, whose cell bodies express vasopressin, oxytocin, and corticotrophic hormone releasing factor. Strong inputs to this nucleus ascend from the midbrain's periaqueductal gray and the (serotonergic) raphe nuclei.

Outputs descending from the periaqueductal gray regulate cardiovascular components of emotional responses. Thelma Lovick (1993), mentioned above, reported how sympathetic premotor neurons of the rostral ventrolateral medulla act as relays in the descending efferent pathway to the sympathetic outflows from the dorsal periaqueductal gray matter (dPAG) which integrates the characteristic "defensive pattern of cardiovascular response that accompanies activation of the midbrain aversive system." She also notes that activity in this pathway can be modulated by a descending pathway which originates in the ventrolateral PAG. Thus, activity in the dorsal system initiates cardiovascular components of aversive/defensive behavior while the ventrolateral system plays an important role in initiating the recuperative phase, sympathoinhibition, typical of recovery from strong emotions.

Along these lines, Nicholas Canteras, in Sao Paulo, Brazil (Motta et al., 2017), suggests that the periaqueductal gray not only regulates the expression of emotion but also that neurons there are involved in "more complex modulation of a number of behavioral responses and work as a unique hub supplying primal emotional tone" to complex aversive and appetitive responses. Of particular relevance, Canteras holds that the PAG is involved in influencing complex forms of defensive responses. In addition, he discusses putative dorsal PAG ascending paths that are likely to convey information related to threatening events to limbic forebrain circuits involved in the processing of fear learning.

A leading neuroscientist, Barbara Jones, of McGill University (Jones and Yang, 1985) followed axons descending from the mesencephalic reticular formation by a technique called tritiated amino acid autoradiography. After microinjections of [³H]leucine, there were labeled axons reaching the medullary reticular formation. Jones' neuroanatomical findings exactly match physiological findings from my lab. MD/PhD student Sandra Cottingham recorded electrical responses from axial (deep back) muscles during combined electrical stimulation of the reticular formation and midbrain central gray. Central gray stimulation facilitated reticular formation-evoked activity in the back muscles of the rat. Electrical stimulation of the central gray lowered the threshold for reticulospinal activation of axial muscles and could maintain firing in these muscles even after the end of a reticular formation train (Cottingham et al., 1987). In this action, reticulospinal neuronal excitation facilitates vestibulospinal effects, and vice versa (Cottingham et al., 1988).

As well, in Jones' results, there were strong ascending projections both to the central thalamus and there were axons running ventrally, past the hypothalamus into the basal forebrain. At the end of this chapter, I will portray the functional importance of a high road from midbrain to forebrain and a low road to hypothalamus and basal forebrain. Jones' findings show that midbrain reticular formation neurons next to the periaqueductal gray (central gray) contribute importantly to both the "roads."

Neurotransmitters. Two well-studied neurotransmitters, dopamine and serotonin, have been implicated in CNS arousal processes for decades. Each implies at least four genes whose appropriate expression and regulation are required: (i) a gene for a synthetic enzyme; (ii) at least one gene coding for a cognate receptor; (iii) a gene for a neurotransmitter re-uptake; and (iv) a gene for chemical breakdown of the transmitter. I will discuss dopamine, followed by serotonin.

Dopamine

Let's start with the basics. Dopamine is synthesized from the amino acid tyrosine by the rate-limiting enzymatic reaction using tyrosine hydroxylase to make DOPA, which is then enzymatically converted into dopamine (Devi and Fricker, 2016a). Two regions in the midbrain contain neuronal groups which are major sources of dopamine signaling: the substantia nigra and the ventral tegmental area. Even now, we do not know why, during development, certain embryonic neurons that will be dopaminergic end up in one of these neuronal groups rather than the other. For discussing generalized CNS arousal, it is sufficient to concentrate on the ventral tegmental area, as the substantia nigra neurons are involved primarily in motor control.

There are five genes coding for dopamine receptors. One subfamily of these receptors, comprising D1 and D5, is expressed at much higher rates than the subfamily D2, D3, D4. All of these five are G-protein-coupled receptors, and the D1 family increases the concentration of cyclic AMP, even as the D2 family has the opposite effect (Devi and Fricker, 2016b).

The neuroanatomy of dopaminergic neuronal projections to the forebrain was opened up with specialized histochemical techniques by a group of neuroscientists at the Karolinska Institute led by Tomas Hokfelt. Projections from ventral tegmental area neurons to frontal and temoral cortex are strong, as are projections to the phylogenetically ancient forebrain, the limbic system. In greater detail, the laboratory of my esteemed neuroanatomy professor at MIT, Walle J. H. Nauta (Beckstead et al., 1979), reported projections not just to basal forebrain areas involved in behavioral reward but also to the central thalamus, to several subnuclei in the amygdala, to the frontal cortex near the midline, and to the cortex adjacent to the amygdala and the hippocampus.

Continuing with the theme that many crucial GA-related neurons have many very short connections as well as very long projections (as from Nauta's lab, above), ventral tegmental area neurons project to the nearby dorsal raphe nucleus (serotonergic, see below) and ventral periaqueductal gray.

Simon and colleagues (1979) did similar work using special tracer application techniques to increase precision, and achieved similar results. Their axonal targets included the prefrontal cortex, the medial part of the lateral septum, the interstitial nucleus of the stria terminalis, the accumbens nucleus, and the olfactory tubercle, as well as the cingulate cortex, the entorhinal cortex, the amygdaloid complex, hippocampus, the accumbens nucleus (associated with behavioral reward), the olfactory tubercle, and the piriform (olfactory) cortex. Thus, ascending axons are presumed to be dopaminergic because they end up in sites where other techniques have shown dopamine terminals. Conversely, Markowitsch and Irle (1981) reported results suggesting that cortical targets of dopaminergic axons may differ from those of non-dopaminergic axons.

Because ventral tegmental area neurons also project down the brainstem to locus coeruleus (which in turn has been shown by Jerome Sutin (McBride and Sutin, 1976) to innervate them reciprocally), there is the possibility of some sort of positive feedback which would produce sudden increase in arousal.

Later work from the premier neuroanatomist Larry Swanson (1982), now at the University of Southern California, yielded results that are in substantial agreement with Nauta and Calas. Loughlin and Fallon's results (1982) added the fact that a given ventral tegmental neuron projects to the left side of the forebrain or the right side, but never both.

Haglund et al. (1979) used an entirely different approach to look at dopaminergic projections to the forebrain. Twenty-four hours after [3H]dopamine ([3H]DA) injections into different parts of the ventral tegmentum, they measured radioactivity recovered in specific forebrain sites. Their results agreed with conventional neuroanatomical studies in showing strong dopaminergic projections to the basal forebrain, the amygdala, and the cerebral cortex adjacent to the amygdala.

Divac et al. (1978) asked a different intellectual question. They wanted to know whether dopaminergic axons from the ventral tegmental area to the prefrontal cortex might converge with projections from the mediodorsal thalamic nucleus. The answer was positive, based on results in three different species. This is important because, at the end of this chapter, I will make a point about how the low road from midbrain toward forebrain and the high road have different types of functional importance. Divac et al. results prove that the two "roads" converge in a cortical region that is crucial for behavioral regulation.

Cooperation among neurotransmitter systems. Cambridge Professor Trevor Robbins has emphasized that different transmitter systems can act jointly to achieve behavioral and psychological functions different than they would if carried out individually (Trofimova and Robbins, 2016). In their review, Chandler and colleagues (2014) agree. For example, Guiard et al. (2008) found that lesioning dopamine neurons using the specific toxin 5-hydroxydopamine decreased the rate of electrical activity of raphe serotonergic neurons by 60 percent. Conversely, selectively destroying serotonin neurons by 5,7-dihydroxytryptamine significantly increased the electrical activity of ventral tegmental area dopamine neurons. The potentials for interactions are clear.

These authors went further to chart similar interactions between locus coeruleus noradrenergic neurons and ventral tegmental area dopamine neurons. During the type of thinking that recalls my development of the GA concept, Cools et al. (2011) were courageous in considering that functions associated with both dopamine and serotonin might result from a single root mechanism. They associate dopamine with behavioral activation (and reinforcement) and serotonin with behavioral inhibition (and aversive processing) – thus, dopamine to seek rewards and serotonin to avoid punishment. Cools and Daw sharply distinguish the well-studied phasic changes in neurotransmission from tonic neurotransmission which they would like to emphasize. Thus, while various dopaminergic, serotonergic, and noradrenergic subsystems may have distinct roles in the modulation of behavior, they can also be seen as acting in cooperative and complementary ways to influence, for example, frontal cortical function.

Inferring functions of ventral tegmental dopaminergic neurons. Important roles for dopamine signaling in the support of CNS arousal have long been widely accepted. Studies during the last 10 years or so tend to strengthen that conviction. One such effort dissected dopaminergic contributions to the arousal-supporting actions of Modafinil, prescribed, according to Jared Young (2009) "for somnolence, shift work sleep disorder and obstructive sleep apnea syndrome" (p. 2663). Modafinil also supports vigilance by our military fighting under unusual conditions and at unusual times on the other side of the world. Young's review offers assurance that dopamine plays a role because, in mice bearing a knockout of the gene for the dopamine transporter, modafinil is not effective at encouraging wakefulness. Pharmacologic and genomic evidence show that both the D1 receptor family (D1 and D5) and the D2 receptor family (D2, D3, D4) participate in the chain of mechanisms by which modafinil supports arousal.

One of the most popular stories about dopamine has to do with behavioral reward. Clearly, projections to nucleus accumbens in the basal forebrain, famously associated with reward phenomena, would fit in with that idea (Han et al., 2017). However, Cambridge Professor Wolfram Schultz has taken the story much farther. He (Schultz, 2016a, 2016b) has focused on dopaminergic neuronal responses to situations where predictions of rewards differ from actual, received rewards. Based mainly on his extensive electrophysiological and behavioral work with monkeys, his conclusion is that "Most dopamine neurons in the midbrain of humans, monkeys, and rodents signal a reward prediction error; they are activated by more reward than predicted (positive prediction error), remain at baseline activity for fully predicted rewards, and show depressed activity with less reward than predicted (negative prediction error)." Further, he has encased his theoretical efforts in economic decision theory, envisioning the animals' behavioral approaches and choices as functions of subjective value, and in its mathematical counterpart, utility (Schultz, 2015).

Scientists value parsimony, i.e., care and economy in the use of assumptions and the application of interpretations. In my discussion of midbrain neuronal dopaminergic function, therefore, I admire the work of Columbia University Professor Jon Horvitz (2000) whose combinations of electrophysiological, neuropharmacological, and behavioral experiments with laboratory rats indicate "that these neurons respond to a large category of salient and arousing events, including appetitive, aversive, high intensity, and novel stimuli." Horvitz connects increased dopaminergic activity with *arousal*. "Dopamine neurons respond to salient and arousing change in environmental conditions, regardless of the motivational valence of that change." This is a more parsimonious depiction of midbrain dopaminergic function than an exclusive focus on reward prediction. After all, one of many ways of rendering a stimulus "salient" would be to associate it with reward! In truth, some of Schultz's more recent results (Stauffer et al., 2016) have taken account of this distinction between salience *qua* salience and reward prediction in reporting that there are at least two components to dopamine responses to reward – an initial, unselective "detection" component that depends on the salience of environmental stimuli, followed by a more specific component that encodes reward value. Most recently, da Silva and Costa (2018) reported that electrical activity of dopamine neurons in the substantia nigra *pars compacta* is necessary for the initiation of movement, as expected for an arousal-related neurotransmitter.

Trevor Robbins (Trofimova and Robbins, 2016) gives us a broader view of dopaminergic neuronal functions supporting CNS arousal. He emphasizes combinations of transmitter contributions and cross-effects between arousal-related transmitters. Dopamine does not serve the "orienting" or the "maintenance" aspects, instead the "dynamical aspects" of behavior. In "action-integration" mode, dopamine facilitates the "physical tempo speed of integration of an action in physical manipulations with objects with well-defined scripts of actions." Even the ability to increase "the preferred speed of speech and ability to understand fast speech on well-known topics, reading and sorting of known verbal material." Every one of these functional assignments must be understood in the context of cooperating transmitters and neuropeptides.

Finally, a caution must be issued against the tendency to highlight, exclusively, the importance of ventral tegmental area neurons in providing dopaminergic support of arousal. The data come in a paper from Clif Saper's lab (Lu et al., 2006). They identified dopaminergic neurons whose apparent activity is correlated with wakefulness by using histochemistry to detect expression of an immediate early gene, Fos, whose molecular signature is often correlated with increased electrical activity. Distinct from the ventral tegmental area, about half of the dopaminergic neurons in the midbrain's ventral periaqueductal gray showed Fos expression during natural wakefulness (but not sleep) and during environmentally induced waking. Damaging these neurons pharmacologically increased sleep. Thus these midbrain dopaminergic neurons near the periaqueductal gray must be added to the groups of cells we consider as important for CNS arousal.

Molecular biology of dopamine cells. Still other dopamine neurons hold great interest for neuroendocrine function and for potential relief from motor disorders. Romanov et al. (2017) used single-cell RNA sequencing to distinguish a considerable number of dopaminergic cell types in the hypothalamus. For instance, their study revealed dopamine neurons that uniquely co-express the Onecut3 and Nmur2 genes, and placed these in the periventricular nucleus and therefore of potential importance for endocrine and behavioral responses to stress and for the management of social behaviors.

Dopaminergic neurons in the substantia nigra are known to be important for staving off Parkinson's disease. Lorenz Studer, M. D. (2012), is leading the charge to produce dopamine neurons from embryonic stem cells as a potential experimental therapy for the treatment of Parkinson's disease. His novel protocols for doing this, including "using an alternative differentiation strategy that is based on deriving midbrain dopamine neurons via a distinct midbrain floor plate intermediate," give him the chance to look ahead toward the possibility of human cell therapy (Studer, 2017). He has shown that such neurons can be cryopreserved prior to transplantation and can be engrafted into the brains of non-human primates. Studer and others emphasize the utility of his approach as opposed to the use of embryonic stem-cell-derived precursor cells as is beginning this year in hospitals in Zhengzhou, China. These Chinese scientists don't know what their engrafted cells will become.

Serotonin (5-HT)

Starting from the basics, once again, serotonin is synthesized from the amino acid tryptophan using the rate-limiting enzyme tryptophan hydroxylase and a second enzymatic conversion to make serotonin (also known as 5-hydroxytryptamine, 5-HT) (Devi and Fricker, 2016a). Surprisingly, there are at least 14 genes that encode serotonin receptors, grouped into at least four subfamilies, each with different biochemical couplings in the downstream neurons (Devi and Fricker, 2016b).

Experiments involving serotonin's relation to arousal have been going on for a long time. More recently, Gordon Buchanan and George Richerson (2010), neurologists at Yale University School of Medicine, launched their experiments knowing that the electrical activity of some serotonergic neurons is stimulated by heightened levels of carbon dioxide and, in addition, that serotonin can stimulate thalamocortical networks. Mice genetically engineered to lack serotonin neurons did not have any arousal response to heightened carbon dioxide. My goal in this section is to explore how serotonin's arousal-related functions are carried out and how to interpret them.

Serotonin is synthesized in neurons close to the midline of the midbrain. They are in the so-called raphe nuclei, where "raphe" comes from the Greek word for "fence" (between the left and the right midbrain). These nuclei supply a rich innervation to the forebrain. My student Lily Conrad et al. (1974) performed an exhaustive study charting axons ascending from the raphe nuclei. The majority of the ascending projections sweep ventrally from the raphe nuclei, then curve rostrally to course through the ventral tegmentum and into the medial forebrain bundle (MFB). Others radiate through the mesencephalic reticular formation (RF) and central gray, turning ventrally at the posterior thalamic border to enter the subthalamus. Important for a point I will make below about a "high road" and "low road," axons from raphe neurons strongly innervate the central thalamus. From the MFB, fibers branch into the hypothalamus, preoptic areas, anterior amygdala, and olfactory tubercle, while some fibers enter the fornix on their way to the hippocampus, or the stria terminalis on their way to the amygdala. Many fibers continue rostrally in the MFB, joining the diagonal bands of Broca to reach the septal nuclei or, further rostrally, the cingulum bundle. Fibers in the cingulum bundle turn caudally around the genu of the corpus callosum, some branching into the cell-free layers of the pregenual cortex. Running caudally, then curving around the splenium, the cingulum bundle projection sprays out into the subiculum and in some cases a projection into the hippocampus is seen. This is an amazing sweep of ascending influences from the raphe.

It is particularly notable that raphe serotonergic neurons have many very short, local projections as well as the long axoned projections just described. As with other systems described in this book, I think that we may be dealing with a scale-free serotonergic network.

What are the molecular and biophysical properties of these raphe neurons of such great influence? Benedict Mlinar, working with Cornelius Gross' unit (2016) at a European Molecular Biology Unit in Italy, recently used a combination of molecular markers and loose-cell-attached electrophysiological recording to bring the characterization of these neurons into the twenty-first century. They found "a wide homogeneous distribution of firing rates, well fitted by a single statistical function" suggesting that, in terms of intrinsic firing properties, "serotonergic neurons in the DRN represent a single cellular population." These serotonergic neurons "exhibited regular, pacemaker-like activity," which might be linked to the functional inferences published by Trevor Robbins, as I cover below.

Inputs. I particularly note that midbrain raphe neurons are addressed by many of the same neurons that send axons to locus coeruleus, especially since some of those neurons are in NGC (highlighted here in Chapter 2) (Lee et al., 2005).

Functions. By far, the most convincing associations of serotonergic neurons with human brain function have to do with depression. From my own theoretical perspective, depression features a devastating loss of arousal regulation. Nautiyal and Hen (2017) face the complexity of serotonergic signaling through 15 or more receptors in several forebrain regions. The best-known means of heightening serotonergic action is to prevent the reuptake of serotonin by the neuron whose synaptic ending just released it. Thus, the drugs in the category Selective Serotonin Reuptake Inhibitors (SSRIs) were developed to treat depression. Mouse studies support this choice. Mice bearing knockouts of the gene for the serotonin transporter, which carries out the reuptake, show depressive-like behaviors. Among patients, a serotonin gene mutation that yields a shorter gene allele and lower levels of the serotonin transporter is correlated with a higher risk of depression.

Extending the serotonergic theory of depression into analyses of which serotonin receptors are involved with depression has been a hard slog. For starts, most of the 15 receptors seem somehow to be involved. Further, it is bewildering that both conventional postsynaptic receptors and autoreceptors (on the neuron that just released the serotonin) must be considered, and that autoreceptors located at different places on the neuron's membrane have different actions. None of this subtlety is particularly surprising to the neuroscientist, but the complexities have required great effort and patience by those working on the problem. Out of all this work it has become clear that the 5-HT1B receptor acting as an autoreceptor is involved, but there is a long way to go.

Taking a wider view of serotonergic function, Trevor Robbins, the Cambridge professor referred to above (Trofimova and Robbins, 2016), emphasizes the importance of serotonergic signaling for more complex mental and behavioral regulations, including the maintenance of alternatives. This is not the initiation of behavior that I spoke about in

Chapters 1 and 2, but "tonic arousal that energizes selected behavioral alternatives whilst also maintaining behavioral inhibition over irrelevant inputs and outputs." In Robbins' view, serotonin cooperates with other transmitters, particularly acetylcholine, to permit *sustained* behavioral activity "using well-defined behavioral elements," including "the ability of an individual to sustain prolonged social-verbal activities." *Mental endurance* depends on serotonin. Relying on results from SUNY Stony Brook Professor Efron Azmitia (2010) and Princeton Professor Barry Jacobs (Jacobs and Fornal, 2010), Robbins distinguishes serotonin's roles from those behavior-initiating functions I highlighted in Chapters 1 and 2, and instead focuses on tonic vigilance and maintenance of activities.

In a most surprising experiment, Steve Flavell et al. (2013) in Cori Bargmannn's lab at Rockefeller, working with an invertebrate, support Trevor Robbins' interpretation of serotonin function. Flavell studies of the worm *Caenorhabditis elegans* focused on the maintenance of discrete behavioral states. Two such states in this tiny worm are called long-lasting "roaming" and "dwelling" states. Bottom line: serotonin promotes dwelling states through a serotonin-gated chloride channel. The rough analogy to Robbins' conclusion from work with mammals is astounding.

High Road, Low Road

As summarized above, some arousal-related axons ascend from the midbrain and dive ventrally as they go forward to the hypothalamus and basal forebrain (the "low road"), while others project straight forward into the central thalamus (the "high road"). Clif Saper's lab at Harvard (Fuller et al., 2011) has emphasized the low road for supporting arousal in rats.

In these lab animals, extensive thalamic lesions had little effect on electroencephalographic (EEG) or behavioral measures of wakefulness. In contrast, animals with large basal forebrain lesions were behaviorally unresponsive and had low-frequency sleep-typical EEG. Saper's experiments indicated that in rats the reticulo-thalamo-cortical pathway may play a very limited role in behavioral or electrocortical arousal, whereas the projection ascending to the basal forebrain may be critical for arousal.

Thus, Saper and his colleagues emphasized roles for basal forebrain in arousal and held that, in rats, thalamocortical systems play little role. However, in human patients, extensive thalamic damage (Caballero, 2010, and see Chapter 8) causes loss of consciousness. The potential roles for extra-thalamic damage in such patients remain to be understood. Importantly, electrical stimulation of the central thalamus can allow a vegetative-state patient to regain consciousness (Schiff et al., 2007).

I propose that both the high road and the low road are important. In species like rats and mice, as well as in humans, the low road serves GA by regulating CNS state through the hypothalamus and basal forebrain. In humans, the high road supports selective attention to sensory stimuli and guided movements.

Chapter 5

Hypothalamus: Low Road

Arousal signals originating in or reaching the hypothalamus are of particular importance because of hypothalamic neurons that regulate several endocrine systems. At least six such systems in the anterior pituitary gland depend on hypothalamic inputs. Hypothalamic oxytocin and vasopressin, important for controlling several body organs, are secreted into the blood through the posterior pituitary gland. Further, hormone-dependent behaviors featuring high CNS arousal, such as sex, stress, and aggression (Chapter 7) depend on hypothalamic mechanisms.

This chapter discusses two generalized arousal (GA) neurochemicals expressed in hypothalamic neurons – histamine and hypocretin (orexin). After that, I will address the biological clock resident in the suprachiasmatic nucleus (SCN) of the hypothalamus, governing sleep–wake cycles. Finally, the idea that arousal signals ascending from the brainstem take a "low road" to regulate the state of the brain and body in lab animals and humans will open into a discussion of large cholinergic neurons in the basal forebrain. These cholinergic neurons have widespread electrophysiological effects in the cerebral cortex (Figure 5.2).

Histamine

Histamine is produced from the amino acid histidine by the enzyme histidine decarboxy-lase. Histamine-producing neurons in the hypothalamus project diffusely throughout the forebrain and brainstem. Their electrical activity is significantly higher during waking than sleeping (when they are inhibited). Working through two receptor types, H1 and H2, they promote waking (Lin J. S. and Haas, 2011; Panula et al., 2015). Histamine is implicated in mechanisms used to make the drug modafinil effective, e.g., in keeping American soldiers alert during long tours of duty (Ishizuka et al., 2012). Conversely, anti-histamines have the side-effect of inducing sleep. Levels of histamine in the brain vary across the 24-hour day, being highest during wakefulness (Lin J. S. and Haas, 2011) and lowest during rapid eye movement (REM) sleep. These data confirm that histamine, produced in a small group of hypothalamic neurons, acts in a major way as an arousal-heightening neurotransmitter. Their electrical activity is significantly higher during waking than sleeping (when they are inhibited). In fact, using the difficult technique of in vivo single cell recordings, J. S. Lin in Lyon finds histamine neurons exclusively active during waking and inactive during sleep.

H1 and H2 receptors do not work in the same way. H1 provides direct excitation of post-synaptic neurons, while H2 action is less direct, working through kinase cascades (Lin J. S. and Haas, 2011). The H3 receptor works the opposite way (Schwartz, 2011; Panula et al., 2015). It feeds back onto histaminergic neurons, inhibits them, and reduces histamine release. Obviously, drugs targeting these receptors selectively become candidates for medical use to treat disorders of waking and sleeping. The histamine H3R antagonist/inverse agonist pitolisant has been introduced to the clinic for the treatment of narcolepsy.

Hypocretins

In 1998, two labs reported the discovery of a gene important for GA – hypocretin (de Lecea et al., 1998) also called orexin (Sakurai et al., 1998). This gene yields two neuropeptides that are expressed specifically in the perifornical area of the hypothalamus. From a 130-amino acid precursor, hypocretin-1 (33 amino acids) and hypocretin-2 (28 amino acids) are derived. These hypocretin neurons receive inputs from many areas of the brain, including the forebrain and the brainstem. In turn, the axons of hypocretin neurons project all over the brain, notably to hypothalamic and brainstem neurons that produce arousal transmitters histamine, dopamine, serotonin, and norepinephrine (reviewed, Boutrel et al., 2010). Thus, according to Lin J. S. and Haas (2011), histamine- and hypocretin-neurons, with their reciprocal interactions, "exert a synergistic and complementary control over waking; the histaminergic system is mainly responsible for cortical activation (EEG) and cognitive activities, while the hypocretinergic system is more involved in the behavioral arousal during waking, including muscle tone, posture, locomotion, food intake, and emotional reactions."

The two hypocretin peptides bind to G-protein-coupled receptors (Chen and Randeva, 2004). Receptor type 1 binds hypocretin-1 with high affinity. Receptor type 2 binds both peptides. The gene products for these receptors can be spliced in more than one way, yielding receptor proteins that differ from tissue to tissue.

Studied with several methods which affirm each other, hypocretin peptides clearly support wakefulness (reviewed, Boutrel et al 2010). This statement, based on the stimulation of light-activated channels by optogenetics, includes waking up from sleep as well as waking up from aesthesia. For example, Adamantidis et al. (2007), working with Luis de Lecea, used an excitatory optogenetic protein expressed under the control of the hypocretin promoter to produce hypocretin neuron-driven sleep to wake transitions. A hypocretin receptor type 1 antagonist greatly delayed these transitions. Matthew Carter and de Lecea (2009b) added the concept that hypocretin actions in the brain reinforce the stability of conscious arousal states. By hypocretinergic axons synapsing in the hypothalamus and brainstem "hypocretins can modulate the arousal network (and) also likely are able to modulate behaviors orchestrated by this network" (p. 42). Optogenetically engineered stimulation of hypocretin neurons caused sleep-to-wake transitions throughout the 24-hour dark–light period (Carter et al., 2009b). Crucially, hypocretins can "maintain stability (of high arousal) at levels outside the normal range and is achieved by varying the internal milieu to match perceived and anticipated environmental demands."

Luis de Lecea's lab (Li et al., 2016) has reviewed the wide distribution of hypocretin axons, notably including projections to other arousal-related cell groups (noradrenergic, dopaminergic, serotonergic), as well as other brain regions. The two hypocretin receptors are found with two different neuroanatomical distributions and have different postsynaptic consequences. For example, Joel Elmquist's lab (Marcus et al., 2001) found hypocretin (OX1)R mRNA in many brain regions including the prefrontal and infralimbic cortex, hippocampus, paraventricular thalamic nucleus, ventromedial hypothalamic nucleus, dorsal raphe nucleus, and locus coeruleus. In contrast hypocretin (OX2)R mRNA was prominent in a different distribution including the cerebral cortex, septal nuclei, hippocampus, medial thalamic groups, raphe nuclei, and many hypothalamic nuclei including the tuberomamillary nucleus, dorsomedial nucleus, paraventricular nucleus, and ventral premamillary nucleus. This difference in receptors may play into differences in the behavioral patterns affected by hypocretins. For instance, Glenda Harris and Gary Aston-Jones (2006) used differential patterns of fos immunochyochemistry activation to infer separate roles for different aspects of behavior: arousal and reward. A related theoretical view would state that one function of a portion of these hypocretin neurons serves to wake the animal (or human) up when the animal (or human) is hungry.

Correlations between hypocretins and sleep–wake balance hold up under a variety of physiological conditions. Yoshida et al. (2001) measured hypocretin-1 levels in the lateral hypothalamus and medial thalamus of freely moving rats. Levels "slowly increased during the dark period (active phase), and decreased during the light period (rest phase)." These variations in hypocretin levels in brain may have something to do with the body's energy homeostasis. Emmanuel Mignot's lab (Nishino et al., 2001) worked with narcoleptic patients and with controls, measuring not only hypocretins but also body mass index and the body fat gene product leptin. As expected, hypocretin-1 was found to be decreased in the narcoleptic patients. Also, leptin in the cerebrospinal fluid and body mass index were significantly higher in patients versus controls, possibly indicating altered regulation of the body's metabolism. Finally, Mignot's lab (2001) used the presynaptic protein synaptophysin in hypocretin neurons to follow synaptic modifications over the 24-hour period. They found circadian rhythmicity in synapse number in hypocretin axons, "regulated primarily by the circadian clock but also affected by sleep deprivation." All of these studies tell us that hypocretin neurons are behaving as you would predict from the summaries of hypocretin function I have summarized above.

If this brief description provides a sketch of normal functions of hypocretins, what are the abnormalities resulting from mutations of genes for hypocretins or their receptors?

Narcolepsy. Neurologist/psychiatrist Emmanuel Mignot (Lin et al., 1999), at the Stanford Center for Sleep Sciences and Medicine, took the lead in discovering the medical importance of the molecular and physiological effects of hypocretins just quoted. Mignot identified a hypocretin receptor mutation that causes narcolepsy in dogs (Lin et al., 1999), and also demonstrated that human narcolepsy is caused by a loss of hypocretin neurons in the hypothalamus (Nishino et al., 2000; Peyron et al., 2000). Indeed, mice with targeted disruption of the hypocretin gene displayed narcolepsy-like episodes: "abrupt cessations of purposeful motor activity associated with a sudden sustained change in posture ... ending abruptly with complete resumption of purposeful motor activity" (Chemelli et al., 1999, p. 440). Over the years, Mignot has anticipated that basic research in his area would yield drug therapies for narcolepsy and insomnia.

In the study referred to above, Lin et al. used positional cloning to identify an autosomal recessive mutation of the hypocretin receptor type 2 gene, leading to the dogs having symptoms like narcolepsy. Then the Mignot lab (Hungs et al., 2001a) focused in on the canine hypocretin receptor locus and came up with two types of mutations associated with narcolepsy. One mutation leads to a single amino acid substitution. This one "associated with proper membrane localization, loss of ligand binding, and dramatically diminished calcium mobilization on activation of the receptor." The other mutation, which skips an entire exon, leads to "an absence of proper membrane localization, and unde-tectable binding and signal transduction." As a kind of genetic control to show specificity, Hungs et al. (2001c) determined that a common preprophypocretin mutation was not associated with narcolepsy, now were there changes in the hypocretin promoter associ-ated with narcolepsy.

In summary, as reviewed by Mignot (Taheri et al., 2002), hypocretin neurons have "dense excitatory projections to monoaminergic centers such as the noradrenergic locus coeruleus, histaminergic tuberomammillary nucleus, serotoninergic raphe nucleus, and dopaminergic ventral tegmental area." Thus, the pattern of hypocretinergic projections fits an overall theme of this book: the high degree of interconnectedness of GA-promoting neurons helps to ensure a well-integrated GA system. Genetic deficiencies causing loss of normal hypocretin neurotransmission causes a sleep disorder, narcolepsy.

As a medical doctor, Emanuel Mignot obviously is interested in the efficient diagnosis and treatment of narcolepsy. In terms of diagnosis, Christensen et al. (2015), in Mignot's lab, got electrophysiological results which suggest that there is no need to wait for a narcoleptic patient to lose postural muscle tone and fall down asleep in order to diagnose the patient's illness. Using the electroencephalograph (EEG) they looked for abnormal sleep transitions and found several examples of abnormal transitions (espe-cially, increased numbers of transitions), for example, from the waking state to light sleep – such transitions were associated with narcolepsy. In terms of therapy, the chal-lenge is to make up for the loss of lateral hypothalamic neurons that produce the neuro-peptide hypocretin or loss of hypocretin receptor function. It might seem obvious that making efficient hypocretin-receptor agonists would do the therapeutic job, but such compounds are still not available for use with human patients (reviewed, Zeitzer et al., 2006; de Biase et al., 2017).

Hormones. The significance of the location of hypocretin neurons, in the hypothala-mus, may be related to the strong endocrine relationships of many hypothalamic cells. Steroid sex hormones can affect hypocretin content in the hypothalamus and hypo-cretin receptor expression. Conversely, hypocretins themselves can stimulate luteinizing hormone release from the pituitary gland under specific endocrine conditions.

My lab used a conjugate of hypocretin with the neurotoxin saporin microinjected into the perifornical region of the hypothalamus of ovariectomized female mice, to cause a highly significant reduction in the number of hypocretin neurons there (Easton et al., 2006). Hormone treatment had no effect on this pharmacologically induced loss. The estrogen effect was revealed when it was combined with hypocretin/saporin: the amount of wheel-running during the dark period of the 24-hour cycle was doubled by subcutane-ous estradiol treatment compared to hypocretin/saporin animals not given hormone. In terms of emotional arousal, hypocretin/saporin reduced the amount of freezing/immo-bility to the fearful context in which the animals had received foot shocks, and estrogen treatment significantly reduced it further. Overall, we concluded that estrogens modu-lated hypocretin effects on some aspects of arousal.

Another endocrine/hypocretin connection was discovered by work in Luis de Lecea's lab, this time regarding corticotrophin releasing factor (CRF) and stress (Winsky-Sommerer et al., 2004). CRF axonal terminals contact hypocretin neurons in the hypo-thalamus and CRF administration in a tissue bath of hypothalamic tissue slices increases firing rates in some hypocretinergic cells. Further, the activation of hypocretin neurons in response to stress was blocked by knocking out the gene for a CRF receptor. It makes sense that hypocretin neurons in the hypothalamus play an important role in maintaining the arousal necessary for adequate responses to stress.

In summary, the neuroscience of the hypocretins and their receptors is progressing rapidly, with importance for both the theory of GA and the medical understanding of narcolepsy.

Suprachiasmatic Nucleus of the Hypothalamus

A leading scholar of the hypothalamic cell group termed a "biological clock," Columbia University Professor Rae Silver (Pauls and Silver, 2016), has analyzed how this cell group gets done its job of coordinating daily rhythms. After all, its individual neurons do now follow the same periods or phases of oscillation, so the question of how the SCN works has presented quite a puzzle. From Pauls' and Silver's tabular summary of this dynamic field of work, one can appreciate the high points of the recent 40 years of work.

The first two clues about this nucleus' function were that visual input from the retina reaches the SCN and that damaging the SCN abolishes daily rhythms of arousal levels. Neuronal firing in this nucleus varies in a circadian manner, even if the nerve cells are being recorded *in vitro*.

Genes connected with circadian rhythms (see section below) are expressed in the SCN and can be influenced by environmental lighting. Crucially, this hypothalamic cell group orchestrates biological clocks elsewhere in the body. In 1996, Silver's lab reported an amazing finding that signals diffusing from a transplanted SCN could regulate behavioral rhythms.

Because of the nice theoretical curves of 24-hour rhythms that are easy to draw, SCN oscillatory function became a favorite topic for neuronal modelers. Heterogeneity among different neurons still, even in 2018, poses a significant theoretical challenge, even including oscillators that are opposite in phase to each other. Neurons in the shell of the SCN function differ from those in its core, but that is not the entire story (Pauls and Silver, 2016).

How do the signals from the SCN travel to other parts of the nervous system? Several ways. First, Deurveilher and Semba (2004) showed that two hypothalamic zones, one immediately beneath the paraventricular nucleus and the other in the dorsomedial hypothalamic nucleus, link the SCN to GA sources such as the locus coeruleus, as well as to the orexin neurons and histaminergic neurons mentioned earlier in this chapter. Second, Alice Luo and Gary Aston-Jones (2009) provided evidence that the SCN projects indirectly to the dopamine producing group, the ventral tegmental area. Further, Aston-Jones showed that some SCN neurons project via the dorsomedial hypothalamic nucleus to the locus coeruleus, and this projection regulates the circadian firing of locus coeruleus neurons. Third, following up these demonstrations, the Saper lab at Harvard Medical School (Vujovic et al., 2015) explored the subparaventricular zone. They reported that different subdivisions of this zone are particularly important for two different rhythms: body temperature and sleep. These zones receive inputs from different parts of the SCN. These subdivisions of the subparaventricular zone have overlapping but distinct axonal targets. And once again the results show the high degree of interconnectness of GA-related systems.

In summary, sleep times and other daily arousal rhythms depend on the outputs from the SCN of the hypothalamus. The links from the SCN to the brainstem reticular formation and thus to the initiation of locomotor activity likely involve several pathways:

through these multiple routes, there are links to the serotonergic and orexinergic systems. These can link, in turn, to the brainstem reticular formation. First, as mentioned, there is a diffusible signal from SCN to neural sites regulating locomotor activity (Silver et al., 1996). The precise targets of this diffusible signal remain to be identified. Second, there is a multi-synaptic pathway to the habenula that seems to be important in regulating locomotor activity (Paul et al., 2011). Third, there is a very extensive set of multisynaptic connections from SCN to numerous brain regions (Morin, 2013). Fourth, there are indirect routes: SCN modulation of hormonal and feeding rhythms influences many hormones that act systemically – at many neural and peripheral loci (Pfaff et al., 2004, principles #14, 15) – to affect activity levels; e.g., ghrelin (LeSauter et al., 2009).

Hormones. Once again, considering hypothalamic neurons, there is evidence of hormonal effects. Ilia Karatsoreos, now at Washington State University, and Rae Silver, at Columbia, reviewed evidence that androgenic hormones "modulate circadian behavior directly" via actions in the SCN by androgen-receptor expressing neurons that lie within the SCN. As well, there is growing recognition of sex hormone effects and sex differences in activity/sleep patterns, both normal and clinically significant.

Mechanisms for these effects are being worked out now. Some relevant data are quoted in Chapter 7, but this hypothalamic chapter focuses on SCN (Mong et al., 2011). Karatsoreos et al. (2011) discovered effects of castration on the SCN expression of circadian clock and other genes. Moreover, intracranial implants of testosterone targeted to SCN restored AR expression in SCN and the normal temporal pattern of circadian running activity (Model et al., 2015). Some of these effects may be mediated by androgen receptors which are localized in SCN neurons that receive direct retinal input (Butler et al., 2012).

Genes. When addressing the "biological clock" in the hypothalamus, it is also natural to open the discussion of genes that participate in the regulation of circadian rhythms. In 1971a, b, Richard Konopka and Seymour Benzer at the California Institute of Technology discovered fruit fly mutants with abnormalities in the daily rhythms of their behavior. Years later, Michael Young (reviewed 2001, 2002) cloned *per* (i.e., period), a gene important to the maintenance of a normal 24-hour rhythm. In Ron Evans' words, humans' "self-sustained time-keeping system is generated and maintained by an endogenous molecular machine, the circadian clock, which is a transcriptional mechanism composed of the transcription factors CLOCK and BMAL and their co-repressors, PER and CRY" (reviewed, Zhao et al., 2014). This "molecular machine" features many genetic feedback loops that help to guarantee its stability. Thus, over more than four decades the genes that contribute to our daily rhythms in GA have been elucidated.

Looking to the future, the questions of exactly how SCN outputs are integrated with other neuronal and hormonal influences on GA remain subjects for new studies.

Sleep State Switching

As a nocturnal animal like the mouse experiences the change from the light period during the day to the dark, the animal goes through the remarkably reliable change in CNS arousal – GA, the initiation of motor behaviors – from very low to very high. About 10 years ago, physicist Jayanth Banavar and I theorized that during this change in behavior the CNS is going through a classical "phase transition" analogous to a "liquid crystal" as it changes from crystalline to liquid (Pfaff and Banavar, 2007). In fact, mice exhibit dynamics that govern the initiation of behavior that can be precisely summarized by power laws

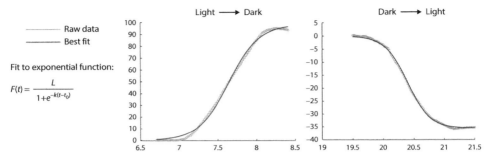

Figure 5.1 The transition from low arousal/activity to high, as the mice pass from the light period of the 24-hour period to the dark, is closely matched by the output of Equation 5.1. Surprisingly, the same equation matches the offset of arousal/activity when the mice pass from the dark period to the light (Rahman et al., 2018). This close match holds true for the individual animals.

which are typical of phase transitions in physics (Proekt et al., 2012). An advantage of this dynamic is that the CNS achieves what a physicist would call "criticality," extreme sensitivity to small changes in the environment for the purpose of initiating useful behaviors. Banavar and I further proposed that *during very low levels of arousal*, the appropriate neural circuits are governed by deterministic chaos in which complicated dynamics are determined by relatively simple equations (e.g., Equation 5.1).

Now, my lab is looking at that transition (Figure 5.1) from the light part of the 24-hour cycle to the dark in mathematical detail (Rahman et al., 2018). Two surprising results have emerged so far. First, the rise in behavioral vigor with increasing arousal can be described by a precise and relatively simple exponential equation.

$$F(t) = \frac{L}{1 + e^{-k(t-t_0)}} \tag{5.1}$$

where L determines the final height of the curve, t the time, and k the slope.

Second, even more surprising, the offset of behavioral activity at the end of the dark period is symmetric to the onset, described by the same Equation 5.1 (Rahman et al., 2018).

How exactly, in terms of neural circuitry, is this phase transition governed? As Clifford Saper, chair of neurology at Harvard Medical School, has pointed out there are occasions when sleeping animals and human beings, obviously more vulnerable to various maladies, must wake up quickly. As in physical scenarios, a faster transition can be achieved if stability up until time zero has been maintained by two well-balanced physical forces pulling against each other (and rapidly adjusted) than by having just one source of influence. In the brain, with respect to sleep–wake transitions, I am convinced by Saper's (2005a, 2005b, 2010) argument – amplifying and clarifying my MIT teacher Walle J. H. Nauta's early suggestion – that two neuronal sources tug against each other in order to regulate sleep–wake transitions. These two are "a sleep-promoting neuronal group, the ventrolateral preoptic area (at the base of the forebrain) and the tuberomammillary nucleus (produces histamine, which wakes us). And during recovery sleep after twelve hours sleep deprivation the amount of slow waves (in the EEG) and the firing of ventrolateral preoptic area neurons both approximately double" (p. 14). As reviewed by Saper, "recordings from ventrolateral preoptic area neurons across the wake-sleep cycle show that their firing rates increase with EEG slow waves." These preoptic neurons increase their firing rates just before or at the transition from waking to (non-rapid eye movement sleep) "and a sharp decrease just before the transition to waking" (p. 11). On the other hand, there are also wake-promoting neurons, the histaminergic neurons in the hypothalamic tuberomammillary nucleus, described above in this chapter. The key point is that the mutually inhibitory connections known to exist between these histaminergic (wake-promoting) neurons and the ventrolateral preoptic (sleep-promoting) neurons enforce well-regulated, rapid transitions between waking and sleeping.

Modern work on the sleep switch opened when the MIT neuroanatomist Walle J. H. Nauta (1946) used lesion techniques to show that damage to the posterior hypothalamus produced a sleepy animal and, conversely, damage to the preoptic area produced a sleepless animal. Nauta proposed that these two regions of hypothalamic and preoptic neurons could oppose each other. Nauta's ideas were sharpened neuroanatomically and conceptually by Cliff Saper. Chronologically, Saper's work on the sleep switch (Sherin et al., 1996) began with the demonstration that neurons in the ventrolateral preoptic area are active during sleep. In this case, the proof of activity did not depend on electrical recording; instead, it used expression on an immediate early gene, *fos*, which triggers expression of many other genes associated with activity. Most importantly, these sleep-activated ventrolateral preoptic neurons innervate the tuberomammillary nucleus of the hypothalamus. Saper et al. (2001) added the observation that "the ventrolateral preoptic nucleus contains GABAergic and galaninergic neurons that are active during sleep and are necessary for normal sleep." In turn, the posterior lateral hypothalamus contains both histaminergic neurons and hypocretin neurons that keep us awake. Saper came up with the sensible idea that these neuronal groups – sleep promoting and wake promoting – inhibit each other. While Sherin's and Saper's paper discussed "stable wakefulness," the actual implication of their ideas accounts for rapid sleep–wake transitions. Saper's lab (Gaus et al., 2002) added that sleep-active ventrolateral preoptic neurons express mRNA for the inhibitory neuropeptide, galanin, in nocturnal rodents and other animals.

All of this work is interesting from a medical and pharmacological point of view. Further, consider leptin, the product of a gene expressed in fat cells, which was cloned by Jeffrey Friedman at Rockefeller University in 1994. Already by 1997, Joel Elmquist and Cliff Saper at Harvard had shown that administration of leptin activates neurons in the hypothalamus, including some that regulate autonomic mechanisms, both parasympathetic and sympathetic neurons. Sleep-switching neurons are also implicated in the mechanisms of action of the drug modafinil, used to keep people awake during unusual situations, such as battle (Scammel et al., 2000). To the point, modafinil increased expression of the immediate early gene Fos in the histamine-producing tuberomammillary nucleus (TMN) and in hypocretin neurons of the lateral hypothalamus.

There is a hormonal connection as well. In our hands (Mong et al., 2003a), estradiol dramatically suppresses expression of a gene that produces prostaglandin D, a somnogen, in the ventrolateral preoptic area. Then, when we (Mong et al., 2003b) used antisense oligonucleotides to reduce the mRNA for prostaglandin-D synthase, specifically in the ventrolateral preoptic area, we produced mice with a heightened arousal state and increased latency to sleep. Following that up, Jessica Mong, now professor at the University of

Maryland Medical School (Hadjimarkou et al., 2008), showed that in females with physiological levels of estradiol, Fos expression – as a sign of neuronal activation – during the light phase of the daily light cycle when mice sleep, was significantly reduced in the ventrolateral preoptic area. Sleep-active neurons were inhibited (and, by the way, wake-promoting histaminergic neurons are activated in the female hypothalamus). And the expression of prostaglandin-D synthase was reduced as well. There were no hormonal effects in males. Then, using telemetry to record the cortical encephalograms of females, Mong could detect a marked reduction in both deep sleep and rapid eye movement sleep when estrogen levels are high. Thus, at least some of the sex hormone effects on GA are routed through the ventrolateral preoptic area.

In summary (Saper et al., 2010), neurons known for decades to be important for sleep, in the ventrolateral preoptic area, "receive reciprocal inputs from many regions implicated in arousal," including, most convincingly, the histaminergic neurons of the tuberomammillary nucleus of the hypothalamus and the noradrenergic neurons of the locus coeruleus. The interactions of the sleep-producing and wake-producing neurons, inhibiting each other, provide mechanisms for sharp sleep–wake transitions.

Low Road: The Lateral Hypothalamus' Medial Forebrain Bundle

At the base of the forebrain, in front of the midbrain, axons which originated in brainstem arousal-promoting neuronal groups sweep past the medial hypothalamus in the so-called "medial forebrain bundle." Large cholinergic neurons in the basal forebrain constitute an important synaptic target of these axons (Zaborszky and Cullinan, 1989; Cullinan and Zaborszky, 1991).

Gritti and Jones (2006) charted how these cholinergic neurons are distributed among neurons using other neurotransmitters, especially GABA. These cholinergic neurons excite cerebral cortical activity in multiple, complex ways. They are spread across four separate nuclear groups (Villano et al., 2017) and, as summarized by Lin and Haas (2011), they "discharge tonically during both wakefulness and paradoxical sleep, can excite cortical neurons directly and suppress the thalamic reticular nucleus oscillation" which generates a "sleepy" EEG. "Basal forebrain cholinergic neurons can relay excitation (e.g., from glutamatergic, noradrenergic, and histaminergic neurons) from the lower brain reticular structures to the cortex." Villano et al. (2017) lay special emphasis on the ability of orexin inputs to excite basal forebrain cholinergic neurons and thereby to increase acetylcholine release in the cortex. There is no doubt that these large neurons are involved in increasing CNS arousal, particularly as manifested by cortical electrical activity.

Villano et al (2017) emphasize the impact of hypocretins released in the basal forebrain on cholinergic neurons lying there. Both hypocretin receptors are expressed there but, as reviewed by Villano, the two may play different roles. For the purpose of this chapter it is important to understand that administering hypocretins into the basal forebrain "excites cholinergic neurons that release acetylcholine in the cerebral cortex and thereby promotes wakefulness."

In general, the number of arousal-related neurons projecting to basal forebrain supports a major theme in this book: the high degree of interconnectness among GA subsystems helps to ensure a well-integrated output. In addition, there is a wealth of anatomical evidence for diverse inputs to BF cholinergic neurons, including from the striatum, frontal cortex, brainstem, lateral hypothalamus, and other neuromodulatory centers (Zaborszky et al., 2012).

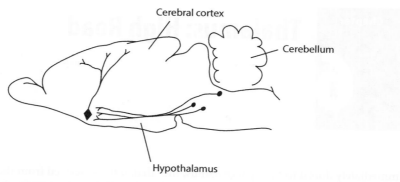

Figure 5.2 Some arousal signals ascending from brainstem norepinephrine, dopaminergic, and serotonergic neurons reach large cholinergic neurons in the basal forebrain. These cholinergic cells send a vast and important array of signals to the cerebral cortex

Basal forebrain cholinergic neurons sometimes work together with co-transmitters. Ma et al. (2017) have reviewed evidence that, in addition to acetylcholine, they can release glutamate or GABA. A similar situation holds for hypocretin neurons, which can release galanin or glutamate. And, again, for histamine neurons, co-transmitters include glutamate or GABA. The precise physiological significance of co-transmitter participation is not yet understood, at least in these cases. In the words of McGill Professor Barbara Jones (2005) "acetylcholine (ACh)-containing neurons discharge during waking, decrease firing during slow wave sleep and fire at high rates during paradoxical sleep in association with fast cortical activity. Neurons that do not contain ACh, including GABA-containing neurons in the basal forebrain and preoptic area, are active in a reciprocal manner to the neurons of the arousal systems." That is, by using juxtacellular recoding techniques Lee and Jones (2005) showed that cholinergic basal forebrain neurons have their highest rates of electrical activity during waking and paradoxical sleep, when high frequencies of electroencephalographic activity are present.

A tremendous amount of molecular work has been put into determining the nature and sequence of transcriptional steps involved in the development of basal forebrain cholinergic neurons (Allaway and Machold, 2017). In these authors' words "All forebrain cholinergic projection neurons and interneurons appear to share a common developmental origin in the embryonic ventral telencephalon." These transcriptional events include, but are not limited to, homeobox gene products, for example, Nkx2.1 (acting relatively early) leading to Gbx-1 and Gbx-2, followed in turn by growth factors such as nerve growth factor (NGF) and brain-derived neuronal growth factor (BDNF).

Summary

The hypothalamus plays importantly into GA mechanisms for two different types of reasons. First, it contains the nerve cell groups that express and transport histamine and the hypocretin peptides. Second, the medial forebrain bundle in the lateral hypothalamus serves ascending arousal-related axons as the route to large cholinergic neurons in the basal forebrain. For GA, this is the low road. The next chapter discusses the high road.

Thalamus: High Road

Immediately dorsal to the hypothalamus, the "thalamus" – derived from the Greek word for "foyer" or entryway – provides the entryway for all the sensory systems (other than olfaction) to the cerebral cortex. According to David Amaral (2000) among the major divisions of the thalamus, for questions about generalized arousal (GA) we must attend to the region called the medial thalamus (aka central thalamus, intralaminar nuclei [pp. 341–3]). Neurons in this region, e.g., the mediodorsal nucleus of the thalamus, receive major inputs from the spinal cord's anterolateral pathway, with signals processed in part by the nucleus gigantocellularis (Chapter 2) and by nuclei in the midbrain (Chapter 4).

Regarding GA, the thalamus constitutes the "high road" to the forebrain. Its position in GA pathways illustrates several themes in this book, as detailed below. The central thalamus gains its integrative power in part from the high degree of interconnectedness of ascending GA-related neurons. It represents the apex of long distance anterior/posterior, longitudinal (A/P, L) integrated systems, whose distributions of connection numbers seem to represent a scale-free system. The largest reticular neurons in the ascending GA system sending the same message over both short and long distances force the integration needed for coherent GA regulation.

High Road: Effects of Thalamic Damage

There is no doubt that damage to the "high road" to the forebrain reduces conscious awareness. Paramedian thalamic damage as caused by a stroke is associated classically with loss of consciousness (Adams et al., 2000; Kumral et al., 2001; Caballero, 2010). In detail, loss of circulation through the posterior cerebral artery can cause major damage to the thalamus, associated with altered states of conscious including sensory loss (Brust, 2000, p. 1308).

According to Harvard neurology professor Clif Saper (2000), damage caused to the pathway through the thalamus "can impair consciousness" (p. 899). Also, it is thought that certain temporal patterns of action potentials in thalamic neurons can cause electroencephalographic patterns typical of sleep. Consistent with this assertion, Lövblad et al. (1997) examined 12 patients with sleep disturbance by MRI. Two distinct groups of patients could be defined: six presenting with severe hypersomnia and six with slight sleepiness. The severely abnormal group had bilateral thalamic lesions; the less severe group, unilateral. Consistent with the behavioral results, localized delta activity in the electroencephalograph may result from a localized thalamic lesion (Gloor et al., 1977). "Unilateral diffuse delta activity appears on the side of thalamic or hypothalamic lesions. Bilateral delta activity results from bilateral lesions of the midbrain tegmentum." Likewise, thalamic damage can be responsible for reduced metabolism in anterior cortical areas (de Falco et al., 1994).

Strokes from occlusion of branches of the posterior cerebral artery often result in somnolence and other abnormalities of the 24-hour wake–sleep rhythm (older literature reviewed, Schmahmann, 2003). For example, in the case (Zavalko et al., 2012) of a 44-year old man with bilateral paramedian thalamic lesions had irregular sleep–wake patterns coupled with prolonged daytime naps. Likewise, Autret et al. (2011) reported that thalamic lesions reduced arousals and caused sleep instability. Mitchell and Kaelber (1967) found that central thalamic lesions were effective in reducing response to pain.

Traditionally the thalamo-cortical axis is believed to be crucial for the maintenance/recovery of consciousness after brain injury, as well as for cortical/behavioral arousal (reviewed, Schiff, 2008). Evan Lutkenhoff from the Monti Lab shows, in a paper now in press in *Annals of Neurology*, that the degree of thalamic atrophy is proportional to a patient's inability to produce voluntary movement; level of arousal was also connected to the degree of atrophy within the basal ganglia (putamen/globus pallidus).

In terms of the thalamus being important for behaviors that require high GA, Joseph Ledoux's lab at New York University (Johnson et al., 2011) has shown that the signal from an auditory stimulus travels to critical neurons in the lateral amygdala via a direct connection from the auditory thalamus. Part of their evidence was derived from the effects of posterior intralaminar thalamic lesions on foot-shock-induced immediate early gene expression in the lateral amygdala. Such lesions reduced the number of activated neurons in the lateral amygdala, leading to the inference that important foot-shock-related information travels through the posterior intralaminar thalamic nucleus to the amygdala (Lanuza et al., 2008).

Pace-Schott et al. (2008, p. 969) say that "Reciprocally interconnected thalamic and cortical neurons form the circuit that are the physiological basis of oscillations" in the cortical eletroencephalogram from the very slow delta rhythms of deep sleep to the high-frequency gamma waves of the alert cerebral cortex. Brainstem ascending arousal systems covered in Chapters 2–4 impact central thalamic neurons with noisy, unpatterned action potentials to disrupt slow oscillatory thalamocortical activity. This set of facts further illustrates a central theme of this book: the high degree of interconnectedness among GA-related neuronal groups (Figure 6.1).

Pace-Schott et al., summarizing the work of David McCormick, Manuel Steriade, and others, speak of the slow, delta waves of sleep arising either from delta-frequency firing of thalamic neurons or via a feedback from the cortex through to thalamic reticular neurons which hyperpolarize thalamocortical projection neurons.

Finally, an expert in the physiology of consciousness, Christof Koch, writing about consciousness, emphasizes the importance of the central thalamus: "Comparatively small bilateral lesions in the inralaminar nuclei can completely eliminate awareness" (p. 1227).

Thus, from several types of evidence, damage to the "high road" reduces consciousness, especially as measured by sensory awareness and attention.

Network Theory

How does thalamic damage cause disorders of consciousness? Since the thalamus provides the high road to consciousness and comprises the termination of long ascending

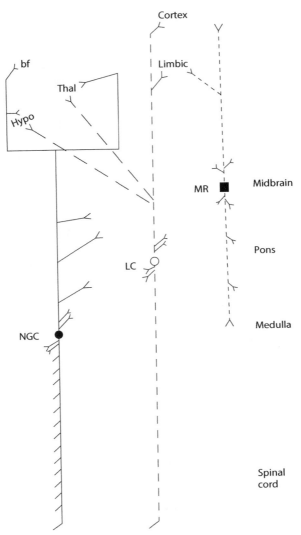

Figure 6.1 Cartoon illustrating the idea of a ladder-like anterior/posterior, longitudinal generalized arousal system that features extremely short connections, medium-length, and extremely long axonal projections. Apparently this may be a scale-free system such that the delivery of the same message from, for instance, an NGC neuron, over such a long range of lengths comprises the very essence of "integration". Nucleus GigantoCellularis (NGC, solid lines _____); Locus Coeruleus (LC, dashed lines - - - - -); Midbrain Raphe nuclei (MR, dotted lines ....). In this partial rendition, the "Low Road" (to the hypothalamus and basal forebrain) and the "High Road" (to the central thalamus) are sketched. Only one side of the system is drawn, but all components are present bilaterally. Other abbreviations: bf, basal forebrain; hypo, hypothalamus; Thal, central (intralaminar) thalamus; Limbic, limbic structures

NGC axons (Tabansky et al., 2018), I consider here some "network theory." If indeed our A/P, L network is scale-free (numbers of connections per neuron in the network obeying a power law) as noted in Chapters 1 and 10, then we are free to theorize about the potential relation to power law GA behavior (see Figure 1.1 and also Proekt et al., 2012).

In neuroanatomical terms, the central thalamus gains its importance in the regulation of CNS arousal from two sets of properties. First, it constitutes a region of convergence for ascending brainstem arousal pathways. Second, its axons spread widely over the cortex, with an emphasis on frontal cortex.

The simple sketch in Figure 6.1 illustrates four points about the A/P, L system that serves GA: first, its ladder-like character; second, the high degree of interconnectivity in GA systems; third, the convergence of ascending arousal systems using different neurotransmitters, on the central thalamus, that is, at a minimum, brainstem arousal systems stimulate central thalamic activity through noradrenergic, glutamatergic, serotonergic, and cholinergic synapses (reviewed, Schiff, 2008); and fourth, the existence of very long distance projections forward from the brainstem, added to plentiful local connections, offers the chance of a scale-free network.

How much farther can we go in applying the emerging network science to GA mechanisms? The statistical physics of network sciences "offers a mechanistic description of a system's dynamics" (Barzel et al., 2015). Issues include a system's controllability (Postfai and Barabasi, 2017), its resilience in the face of "internal failures and environmental changes" (Gao et al., 2016), and a variety of other factors (reviewed, Liu and Barabasi, 2016; Bassett and Sporns, 2017). It appears that controlling our GA system through several hubs would be ideal, energetically (Barabasi, 2015).

Nevertheless, I would interpose a caution. Most network theorists deal with much simpler systems than the brain. In particular, binary digits are their favorites. Therefore, taking results from network science and simply applying them, *pari passu*, to neuroscience would be a dangerous route to take.

Neurophysiology. Some of the ways in which the central thalamus contributes to arousal regulation have been studied with neurophysiological methodology. As compared to the neuroanatomy discussed above, the neurophysiological stories are complex and still evolving. Here I cover a small number of the major themes.

A central point: Cornell neurology professor Nicholas Schiff has hypothesized that activation of a thalamic/cortical/basal ganglia "mesocircuit" plays a central role in the ability of central thalamic stimulation to help a high-end vegetative state patient recover awareness (see below). Schiff's mesocircuit finds its basis in data reviewed, for example, by Joel and Weiner (1994) that demonstrated circuits among the thalamus, frontal cortex, and subcortical motor control regions called the basal ganglia. As well, Groenewegen and Berendse (1994) described central thalamic nuclei sets of connections to different parts of the cerebral cortex and striatum. They reported that "the targets of the thalamocortical and thalamostriatal projections of a given nucleus are interconnected through corticostriatal projections."

One major theme in this area of neurophysiology concerns rhythmic activity in thalamus and cortex, likely achieved in part by feedback from cortex to thalamus. Blumenfeld and McCormick (2000) studied this question using thalamic neurons not in the central thalamus. They constructed an electronic circuit intended to stand in for corticothalamic activity. "With one corticothalamic stimulus per thalamic burst, 6–10 Hz oscillations resembling spindle waves were generated. However, if the stimulation was a burst, the network immediately transformed into a 3–4 Hz paroxysmal oscillation." The work, initially planned to reveal the basis of abnormal cortical activity, has wider application. Because of increased activity in nearby GABAergic perigeniculate neurons, the authors went on to show that signaling through GABA(A) and GABA(B) receptors in response to corticothalamic input patterns help to regulate oscillation frequency of thalamocortical network. This work is of central importance for understanding the state of forebrain electrical activity.

Closely related is the work of Fogerson and Huguenard (2016), who argued that thalamic oscillators, associated with sleep and anesthesia, are under both local and global control. While they were interested in protecting against pathological electrophysiological waveforms, their analyses apply to normal conditions as well.

Zagha and McCormick (2014) emphasized the role of potassium currents in both thalamic neurons and in cortical neurons influenced by thalamic inputs. Closing certain potassium channels would heighten electrical excitability by depolarizing these neurons. Such potassium current closure could, for example, explain the change in cortical electrical activity from deep sleeping to waking. Potassium conductances can be decreased by arousal-related transmitters such as norepinephrine, histamine, and serotonin, as well as by acetylcholine released from the synaptic terminals of basal forebrain neurons. McCormick sees this as an important phenomenon in thalamic neurons and in pyramidal neurons in the cortex.

As mentioned above, the work of Blumenfeld and McCormick implicated the inhibitory neurotransmitter GABA in the regulation of oscillatory activities in thalamocortical systems. Brown and McKenna (2015) insist that "GABA is not purely a sleep-promoting neurotransmitter." Certain GABA neurons have their highest frequencies of action potentials when a cortical electroencephalogram shows very fast rhythms. As well, note that GABA neurons in the thalamic reticular nucleus are particularly important in the thalamus for their relation to "sleepy" EEGs. These thalamic reticular nucleus GABA neurons show "a high expression of T-type voltage-dependent Ca^{2+} channels whose activation shapes the output of the thalamus" Leresche and Lambert (2017). So in the thalamus and projecting to the thalamus we do indeed see sleep-active GABAergic neurons, but we also see GABA neurons "which disinhibit and synchronize the activity promoting the fast EEG rhythms typical of conscious states" (Brown and McKenna, 2015).

Development. Finally, we have not touched on developmental mechanisms that produce the thalamic networks involved in GA (reviewed, Garel and López-Bendito, 2014; Gezelius and López-Bendito, 2017). Early stages of thalamic development employ well-recognized Sonic hedgehog (ventralizing) and Wnt signaling pathways. In general, traditional means of patterning homeodomain transcription factors are employed with the discoveries about patterns of expression, for example, that Dbx1 is expressed in caudo-dorsal thalamus, while Olig2 has a complementary rostro-ventral pattern of expression. One interesting fact is that GABA neuronal populations during development consist of intrinsic inhibitory interneurons supplemented by large numbers of GABA neurons which invaded from neighboring structures. By and large, these discoveries have been driven by unbiased microdissections and microarrays, simply looking for patterns of hox gene expression. No principles of thalamic development have emerged. Regarding thalamic outputs, the array of thalamocortical axons comprises glutamatergic projection neurons following gradients of axon guidance molecules and axon/guidepost cell interactions. These developmental mechanisms, which will determine thalamocortical signaling, obviously provide attractive subjects for further experimentation.

Regarding network theory, if NGC neurons (Chapter 2) comprise a very important hub in the circuit, do we need to worry about massive instability of the arousal circuitry if NGC neurons are damaged? I think not, because GA regulating properties have been ascribed to pontine reticular neurons (Chapter 3) and Marshall Devor's lab (Minert et al., 2017) have recently discovered midbrain neurons essential for the maintenance of anesthesia. Therefore while I call NGC neurons the "master cells" for GA, it is recognized that other hubs (nodes) in arousal circuitry can participate in a manner that fosters network stability.

Stimulation

Since we knew of the 2007 successful work on central thalamic stimulation by Nicholas D. Schiff, MD (see below), in 2008 on behalf of my graduate student Amy Wells Quinkert, we wanted to ask about improving behavioral results of thalamic electrical stimulation by optimizing the temporal patterning of the stimulation pulses (Quinkert et al., 2010). I thought about what kinds of temporal patterning of action potentials our stimulation would be trying to emulate. That is, if it is true that informational content of neural responses is irrelevant to the application of this technique or if the importance lies strictly in the frequency of stimulation, then the current standard clinical practice of choosing the proper frequency, amplitude, pulse width, and stimulation duration is valid and sufficient. If, on the other hand, important informational content is in the temporal pattern of pulses and not just the values of these electrical parameters, it would stand to reason that appropriately patterned stimulation trains might more effectively mimic and substitute for normal neural input.

Over the years, large numbers of theories of the neural coding have tried to answer the classic question of the pattern of neuronal cell responses: neuroscientists observe that neurons fire in particular patterns that can change with stimuli, but do these patterns carry informational content? There are many examples of physiologically relevant temporal patterns, especially in sensory systems, and of how neuronal circuits can use temporal patterning to relay information about changing stimuli. If GA systems are as sensitive to temporal patterning of neuronal responses as sensory systems, then deep-brain stimulation (DBS) to increase GA may also be responsive to different temporal patterns.

In particular, I was impressed with the amplifying power and adaptability of certain nonlinear systems. Deterministic chaotic temporal patterns can result from at least eight equations (Cohen, 1995). I noted that chaotic systems have the potential to exhibit diverse behaviors. In particular, the exquisite sensitivity of chaotic systems to tiny perturbations is a powerful means of directing the trajectories in useful ways. The nonlinear dynamics of deterministic chaos provide exponential amplification of intrinsic fluctuations. The logistic equation lays out the step by step changes in a dynamic system:

$$X_n = RX_{n-1}(1 - X_{n-1}) \qquad (6.1)$$

I chose the logistic equation for its attractive mathematical simplicity and used its temporal series to generate two nonlinear patterns, Nonlinear1 (NL1) and Nonlinear2 (NL2), and the conventional pattern, Fixed Frequency (FF) (Quinkert et al., 2010). Medial thalamic stimulation raised behavioral activity by three separate measures (a count of twitching movements, locomotion, and total activity counts). To the point, for any given behavioral measure, the magnitude of the behavioral increase during and after stimulation depended on the temporal pattern of pulses used. The same result obtained for activation of the cortical electroencephalograph.

It was not the case that the nonlinear temporal patterns of stimulation *always* produced bigger effects than conventional fixed-frequency stimulation. Therefore, Quinkert and I (2010, 2012) started a new set of experiments in which we also included a temporal pattern of randomness as determined by a true random number generator that takes atmospheric noise measurements to generate three thousand uniformly distributed numbers. As expected higher frequencies and higher amplitudes of stimulation tend to produce larger increases in the initiation of motor behaviors. Surprisingly, motor activity increased more with stimulation during the daily light phase than during the daily dark phase. The main result of the study was that behavioral responses to fixed frequency stimulation are not the same as responses to truly random or chaotic stimulation. We do not know exactly how temporally patterned stimulation may affect neuronal circuit dynamics important for CNS arousal.

Mathematician Daniel Keenan followed up the Quinkert et al. work (Keenan et al., 2015). Through his efforts a method was developed to compare the activity in the stimulation interval to that in neighboring intervals, in a manner consistent with the inherent local stationarity of mouse motor activity, which is highly influenced by light and dark. His methods, utilizing piecewise stationarity, allowed one to calculate statistics of motor activity over a segment of time, and, most importantly, to obtain accurate and justified standard errors for those statistics, again for an individual animal. The methods then allowed one to combine results across individual animals, reaching the level of desired inference (drawing conclusions based upon the full data). Besides confirming and extending the Quinkert results – the central thalamic stimulation really works – he was able to derive more information about exactly what changed during central thalamic stimulation. It turns out that it is two-dimensional (2-D) movement, not straight 1-D movement that strongly differs between light and dark and that responds to central thalamic stimulation. Thalamic stimulation in the light initiates a manner of movement – 2-D movement – that is more commonly seen in the (non-stimulated) dark.

Besides investigating basic mechanisms of GA, an important reason for doing central thalamic stimulation is to deepen our understanding of therapeutic maneuvers that may resolve certain disorders of consciousness following traumatic brain injury. In new work (Tabansky et al., 2014) my lab prepared mice with closed-head multiple traumatic brain injury (TBI) and found that, compared to controls, the TBI mice showed decreases in the motoric aspects of GA, as measured by automated, quantitative behavioral assays. Further, we found that temporally patterned DBS can increase GA and spontaneous motor activity in this mouse model of TBI. This arousal increase is input-pattern-dependent, as changing the temporal pattern of DBS can modulate its effect on motor activity. Finally, an extensive examination of mouse behavioral capacities, looking for deficits in this model of TBI, suggests that the strongest effects of TBI in this model are found in the initiation of any kind of movement.

In addition, Daniel Herrera, working with Nicholas Schiff (Shirvalkar et al., 2006), reported that central thalamic stimulation at a high frequency (100 pulses per second) enhanced rat cognitive performance. Stimulation almost doubled the performance of the animals to do novel object recognition. Behavioral improvement – a higher percentage of correct choices of the novel object – was accompanied by widespread cortical activation as measured by expression of the immediate early gene c-fos.

Meanwhile, the Schiff laboratory (Baker et al., 2016) worked with healthy non-human primates using electrodes which offered sites, individual or in combination, of central thalamic stimulation. By using their novel electrode design to orient and shape the field of central thalamic stimulation, they could show that such stimulation "improves performance in visuomotor tasks and is associated with physiological effects consistent with enhancement of endogenous arousal." Re-establishing arousal regulation is important because it would support cognition in seriously brain injured patients. High arousal and motivation at the beginning of a long experimental session which eventually would wane. Likewise, the nature of the thalamic stimulation effect changed as each experimental session wore on, beginning with a decrease in reaction times which disappeared over time. Correlated with behavioral improvements, high frequency local field potentials in frontal cortex/striatum were increased by thalamic stimulation and low frequency potentials were decreased.

While improved task performance and optimal arousal regulation constituted straightforward results of this comprehensive study, Baker et al. also noted shifts in motivational and attentional – one might also say emotional – states that caused them to refer to linkages to autonomic processes related to locus coeruleus. Gary Aston-Jones' and Jonathan Cohen's work on this subject was cited in Chapter 3. In any case, the Baker et al. study demonstrated that central thalamic stimulation "may generalize as a therapy for select SBI patients suffering from the persistent cognitive deficits resulting from serious brain injury."

In fact, the early Schiff et al. (2007) study established proof of principle that central thalamic stimulation can elevate arousal and behavioral performance in a high-end vegetative-state patient, the "minimally conscious state." Schiff's initiative was motivated, in part, by previous work that showed a surprising degree of "preservation of large-scale cerebral networks in patients in the minimally conscious state (MCS), a condition that is characterized by intermittent evidence of awareness of self or the environment. These findings indicate that there might be residual functional capacity in some patients that could be supported by therapeutic interventions." For example, with respect to language-related tasks, responses in the auditory cortex of normal volunteers are much larger for regular spoken narratives than when those narratives are presented backwards, as time-reversed linguistically meaningless stimuli. Minimally conscious state patients' auditory cortex recordings showed the same reduction in response to the time-reversed recordings (Schiff et al., 2005).

The 2007 trial involved a patient who had remained essentially unconscious for more than 6 years. Pre-surgical baseline evaluations confirmed that the patient was in a "minimally conscious state." Under anesthesia, two electrodes each with four contact points of stimulation available were lowered with precise surgical technique into the central thalamus in such a way as to maximize coverage of different subnuclei. "Stimulation produced acute changes in arousal including increased heart rate, well-sustained eye opening and rapid bilateral head-turning to a voice." After several stimulation sessions, the patient tried to name objects and began to make arm movements that "involved social gestures."

As the study went on, there were improvements in the Coma Recovery Scale scores by the patient, and there were "longer periods of eye opening and increased responsiveness to command were reflected in increased Arousal scores." After 143 days in this clinical trial "the patient showed the first instances of functional object use" and intelligible verbalization.

The clinical trial proceeded with stimulation-on periods alternating with stimulating-off periods. The most exciting result to me, as a non-clinical reader, was, over time, the increasing *carryover* of behavioral improvements – increased awareness, command following, etc. – from stimulation-on to stimulation-off. This alone suggested to the optimist that additional well-run trials in the future might garner lasting benefits of relatively brief periods of central thalamic stimulation.

The analysis used a statistical logistic regression approach to show the significance of the effect of central thalamic stimulation on the patient's behavior. Smith et al. (2009) went a step further to do a Bayesian statistical analysis, in which probabilities of current events are estimated given knowledge of the existence of foregoing events. Smith's approach is one used for discrete dynamical systems, for which a state space comprises a set of all the input, output, and state values which a process can assume. Smith's reanalysis, besides simply extending Schiff's paper, offers the possibility of suggesting new central thalamic stimulation strategies to optimize therapeutic efficacy.

Schiff et al. felt that mechanisms for the behavioral improvements might depend on projections from the central thalamus to the frontal cortex (as well as the basal ganglia). His theoretical proposals (Schiff, 2009) have two types of implications. First, in general, he conceived the nature of the recovery processes: their probabilities and their mechanisms. Second, in particular, he wanted to be able to account for a surprising development in which zolpidem, a hypnotic agent that potentiates inhibitory GABA receptors, counterintuitively "improved behavioral responsiveness in some severely brain-injured patients." His resulting theoretical model of recovery of consciousness proposes the following "*mesocircuit*," meaning a circuit which is more encompassing than a local microcircuit, but which does not comprise a whole-brain model. According to Schiff's theory, central thalamic stimulation activates the cerebral cortex widely, importantly including frontal cortex, as well as parietal, occipital, and temporal cortex. It also stimulates activity in subcortical motor control circuits in the striatum of the forebrain. Crucially, the feedback from the striatum to the thalamus includes two inhibitory synapses in a row, such that zolpidem's inhibitory effect on the second inhibitory synapse effectively *disinhibits* normally high levels of thalamic activity. In this way, Schiff's theory can explain the paradoxical effect of zolpidem.

Further, central thalamic stimulation, this time in the mediodorsal nucleus, by optogenetic techniques is reported to amplify cortical connectivity (Schmitt et al., 2017). Mice were subjected to lower frequencies or higher frequencies of stimulation to guide them to attend to vision or audition, respectively. Enhancing central thalamic excitability improves behavioral performance, but the more surprising claim relates to local prefrontal cortex connectivity. This connectivity was measured by additional stimulation and recording within prefrontal cortex, and the data show that central thalamic stimulation more than doubled intra-prefrontal responses to intra-prefrontal stimulation.

A brief paper in Brain Stimulation (2016) by Martin Monti at UCLA offers the possibility that non-invasive ultrasonic acoustical stimulation aimed at the thalamus, delivered as low-intensity pulses, could have a therapeutic effect in a brain-injured patient. An unconscious young man who had suffered severe brain injury in a traffic accident was administered 10 sonication with a pulse repetition frequency of 100/second, each lasting 30 seconds and separated by 30 second intervals. The transducer presenting the sound was located over relatively thin bone on the right side of the temporal cortex and was aimed at the thalamus. After this treatment, the patient did better at following commands, making other motor responses and vocalizing. Three days later, the patient did even better, with "full language comprehension." The authors state that for this one-subject study, "we currently cannot tell whether the observed effects are causally linked to the sonication or whether the patient spontaneously, and serendipitously, emerged from a state of disordered consciousness." For my part, I do not understand the physical mechanisms by which ultrasonic pulses from outside the skull would have the desired neurophysiological effects in the central thalamus, which is in the very middle of the brain.

Monti et al. (2015) also employed the obverse approach, namely, using functional magnetic resonance imaging (fMRI) to detect signs of neuronal activity consistent with cognitive processing in a vegetative state or in the high end of that condition, the "minimally conscious state." Three of eight patients in a vegetative state showed significant activations in the fMRI consistent with the neural activity relevant to the task presented by the physician. Editorial comments on this paper by expert neurologists Serge Goldman (Brussels) and Nicholas Schiff (Cornell, New York) made two points about these and other results in the Monti et al. paper. First, clinical observations of patients with brain injuries "often cannot discriminate large differences in underlying integrative brain function." Second, conversely, "sophisticated functional neuroimaging techniques can fail to identify the capacity to deploy high-level integrative brain functions in patients in whom this capacity appears indisputable on bedside examination."

The broadest point to be made is that in experimental animals and in patients with disorders of consciousness, stimulation of the "non-specific" central thalamus, the intralaminar nuclei, can elevate behavioral performances that depend on GA. This is the high-road serving GA.

Resting State Networks. It is tempting to draw into this discussion the exciting and provocative results from the neurology laboratory of Marcus Raichle at the Washington University School of Medicine. Raichle and colleagues call attention to the fact that the overwhelming preponderance of brain activity is intrinsic, that is, largely independent of overt behavior (Raichle 2001, 2010). Although the physiological functions of this intrinsic activity remain to be determined, accumulating evidence suggests that intrinsic activity does not primarily represent stimulus-independent thoughts (Lauman et al., 2017). Because intrinsic activity is temporally correlated within widely distributed functional systems at all times, even when subjects are quietly resting, the associated topographies currently are known as "resting state" networks (RSNs). Among the RSNs are functional systems associated with somato-motor function, specific senses (visual, auditory), and attention (Fox et al., 2006). Technical insight into the sources of intrinsic signals and warnings about over-interpretation can be found in Snyder (2016).

One RSN discovered entirely as a consequence of functional neuroimaging is the default mode network (DMN). The DMN includes the medial prefrontal cortex, the posterior cingulate cortex, and the lateral parietal cortex, and has representation as well in the cerebellum (Buckner et al., 2011). Cognitive functions assigned to the DMN include recollection, prospection, and theory of mind (Buckner et al., 2008; Nyberg et al., 2010; Jack, 2011). In the present context, it should be noted that reduced activity within the DMN has frequently been reported as a correlate of disorders of consciousness (DOC) regardless of etiology, e.g., post cardiac arrest (Norton et al., 2012), sedation (Fiset et al., 1999), and absence seizures (Laufs, 2012). The DMN is so named because its activity typically decreases during performance of goal-directed tasks (Shulman et al., 1997) while activity in sensory, motor, and attentional areas typically increases. This "push–pull" relation is reflected also in the resting state. Thus, intrinsic activity within the DMN and the "task-positive" system tends to fluctuate in anti-phase (Fox et al., 2005).

Other labs (Doria et al., 2010) followed up these observations by asking whether default mode networks arise as a consequence of experience. To test this idea, they recorded from the brains of infants born prematurely, before the normal term of pregnancy. By the time that a normal full-term birth would have been expected, Doria et al. were able to identify default mode networks, activity that had emerged during the third trimester of pregnancy. Thus, the available evidence indicates that RSNs are present at birth (Smyser et al., 2010). Raichle's lab (Vincent et al., 2007) could also detect default mode activity in the brains of anesthetized monkeys, proving that RSNs are not limited uniquely to the human brain, or, indeed, the waking state.

All of this work on intrinsic activity was done with blood oxygenation level dependent (BOLD) functional magnetic resonance imaging (fMRI). What about the electrical activity as the bases of those BOLD signals? (reviewed by Snyder, 2016). Two labs, using different methods for recording electrical signals from the cortex, picked up the correlations in electrical activity expected across the brain regions from several years of recording BOLD signals (He et al., 2008; Brookes et al., 2011). In addition to confirming the very existence of default mode networks, these results comprise one step toward understanding their underlying cellular mechanisms.

Implicit in some of the work on intrinsic activity has been the hypothesis that fMRI activation in cortical area A correlated with activation in cortical area B occurs because A sends axonal projections directly to B. Horney et al. (2009) tested this idea by achieving high spatial resolution results – the cortical results were divided into 998 separate regions – with two methods. One was the fMRI approach used previously. The other method approached the problem of discerning direct structural connections by using diffusion spectrum imaging tractography, an MRI technique that depends on the fact that in lipid-laden bunches of neuronal axons, water molecules cannot move at equal rates in all directions. Horney et al. found that cortical regions bound by significantly correlated fMRI results did not necessarily have direct structural connections. Therefore, default mode network must depend, in some cases, on indirect axonal projections (e.g., A to C to B).

Fornito et al. (2012) used a different angle of approach to studying RSNs. They interpreted the anti-correlation between task-related networks and default mode as "competitive interactions." Even though several lines of evidence support the sharp distinctions between default mode and task-related systems, Fornito et al. sliced and diced the data in novel ways, with a variety of statistical network analyses. They came away with the conclusions that default mode regions in some cases "cooperate" with sub-components of task-related systems. Further, default mode networks were subdivided into core and "transitional" modules. The key word seems to be "context," a set of undefined features of the environment and behavioral sequence, and its dynamic contribution to the statistical relations between default mode and task-related brain regions. Perhaps part of the definition of "context" lies in the data of Wei Tang and Steven Stufflebeam (2017), who explored "how dynamic connectivity between two regions affects the neural activity within a participating region." They observed changing relations among different parts of the default mode network that depended on the amplitude of fluctuations at different frequencies across the EEG spectrum. They infer "dynamic relationships between local activity and coupling dynamics of a network". Regarding "context" whether this conclusion represents an answer or simply pushes the question back one step remains to be determined.

Now, I wonder how default mode networks may be related to the mesocircuit theorized by Nicholas Schiff (2009) to account for certain incidences of functional recovery from traumatic brain injury. Bonnelle et al. (2012) recorded electrical activity of the cortex of brain-injured (compared to control) subjects during performance of a task that requires the subject to inhibit a learned response that has already been initiated. These trials "require a switch from relatively automatic to highly controlled behavior." They found that efficient inhibition was associated with "rapid deactivation within parts of the default mode network." This deactivation did not occur as reliably in the brain-injured patients, a failure which the authors attribute to damage to a different network they call a Salience Network, responsible for several aspects of cognitive control.

Whether Raichle's analyses of cortical activity shed light on the type of electrical activation required for recovery from traumatic brain injury, or not, presents an intriguing question remaining to be answered.

Summary

Concern over the severe neurological and psychological effects of central thalamic damage can now be offset by hope for progress in the thalamic stimulation techniques intended to restore normal forebrain function. Pathways into and out of central thalamus comprise the "high road" toward the maintenance of GA that functions in parallel with the "low road" through the hypothalamus and basal forebrain covered in the previous chapters. Figure 6.1 illustrates the ladder-like character of the A/P, L system that serves GA, also, the high degree of interconnectivity in GA systems. I noted the convergence of ascending arousal systems using different neurotransmitters onto the central thalamus. And the existence of very long-distance projections forward from the brainstem, as well as the plethora of local connections, offer, theoretically, the chance of a scale-free GA network.

The possible relation of Schiff's "mesocircuit" hypothesized to carry the therapeutic effects of central thalamic stimulation to RSN remains to be determined.

This chapter and the preceding chapters have brought GA networks from the myencephalon (medulla), through the metencephalon (pons) to the mesencephalon (midbrain) and diencephalon (hypothalamus and thalamus). Chapters 7 and 8 switch to the analyses of neural states and behavioral functions which illustrate the roles for GA in behaviors that require high states of arousal (Chapter 7) and neural states that manifest very low levels of arousal (Chapter 8).

High Arousal

Some behaviors reveal high levels of generalized arousal (GA) in their performance and, moreover, require high levels of GA for their execution. This chapter offers three examples of such behaviors: aggression, fear, and sex.

Aggression

As described by Stephen Maxson (in Nelson, 2006, pp. 9–13), display of aggression in mice involves a degree of alertness, strength, and speed of muscular effort that would require high GA. In cats, defensive and offensive patterns, including "rolling on the ground trying to get a good grasp on the other's chest, while kicking their hind legs into the belly of the opponent" (p. 13), similarly display high GA. With aggression, senses must be alert to danger. The body must be prepared for the energy expenditure required by intense fighting.

History. More than 50 years ago, Walter Hess, a physiologist working in Zurich, discovered that electrical stimulation of neurons in certain parts of the hypothalamus or midbrain could cause cats to act angry, or aggressive. He won the Nobel Prize for that work. John Flynn followed it up in an interesting way. A retired priest, Flynn, became a professor at Yale and extended Hess' work by showing that stimulation of different parts of the hypothalamus caused varying aggressive responses. Electrical pulses delivered to the medial part of the hypothalamus caused a cat to act enraged, while stimulation of the lateral hypothalamus led to what Flynn called a "quiet, stalking attack."

Work has continued along these lines, showing repeatedly that stimulation of certain neuronal groups can rapidly produce attack behaviors. In the words of Rutgers Professor Thomas Gregg (2003), "the dorsal and rostral periaqueductal gray is the organizing center for the orchestrated expression of all the behavioral components of the defensive rage response." Recently, Han et al. (2017) reported that optogenetic stimulation of the "central amygdala of mice elicited predatory-like attacks upon both insect and artificial prey. Coordinated control of cervical and mandibular musculatures, which is necessary for accurately positioning lethal bites on prey, was mediated by a central amygdala projection to the reticular formation in the brainstem. In contrast, prey pursuit was mediated by projections to the midbrain periaqueductal gray matter" consonant with the results of Gregg. Lesions of amygdala or central gray each had the opposite effects from those with stimulation.

Genes. Randy Nelson's more recent work on aggression surprised us all because instead of studying regular, conventional neurotransmitters, or the kinds of hormonal influences mentioned below, he used a transmitter which is actually a gas, nitric oxide

(Bedrosian and Nelson, 2014). When he knocked out a gene that produces nitric oxide, he produced mice that attack fast and often. Likewise, when he treated mice with a drug that inhibits that nitric-oxide-producing enzyme, the mice were extremely aggressive.

Work in my lab also showed that we could draw causal connections between the expression of specific genes and aggressive behaviors. Having discovered hormone receptors in the brain, I wanted to chart the behavioral consequences of knocking out genes coding for these receptors. And the connections between these genes and aggressive behaviors are different between males and females. For example, Sonoko Ogawa, in my lab (1998a, b, 2004), determined that knocking out the gene for an estrogen receptor *raised* aggressive behaviors by females, but *lowered* aggressive behaviors by males. Next, Masayoshi Nomura (2002), also in my lab, studied a different nuclear hormone receptor and discovered that knocking out this gene in males caused especially high aggression only just after puberty, which maps on to the tendency in humans for murder rates by males to peak between the ages of 13 and 30.

Our work with gene knock-outs leads directly to Cal Tech Professor David Anderson's work, which has taken the molecular analysis of aggression in a new direction. First, Dayu Lin, then working with Lin Anderson (2011), used brief pulses of light transmitted to the hypothalamus through optical fibers to stimulate activity in ventromedial hypothalamic neurons that had been infected with a special viral vector that permits light to be translated into action potentials. Such optogenetic stimulation "elicited a rapid onset of coordinated and directed attack" (p. 223) toward an intruder.

Then Anderson and his team went on to identify exactly which type of ventromedial hypothalamic neurons could carry the effect of optogenetic stimulation into attack behavior. By designing a viral vector dependent on the neuron with estrogen receptors, they could show that neurons expressing the gene for an estrogen receptor, when activated, caused the attack behavior. Nearby ventromedial hypothalamic neurons, not expressing estrogen receptor, did not work. The more optical stimulation onto these virus-carrying receptor-expressing neurons, the more attack.

In Anderson's words, "recordings from VMHvl during social interactions reveal overlapping but distinct neuronal subpopulations involved in fighting and mating." On the one hand, I am reminded of the thinking of Nobel-winning ethologist Niko Tinbergen when he talked about "action specific energies," i.e., motivational forces that might be directed toward one natural behavior sequence of another, e.g., sex versus aggression. On the other hand, after all, males of several species must defend their territories in order to attract females.

Generalized CNS Arousal. Klaus Miczek et al. (2004) reviewed effects of neurotransmitter-related drugs on aggressive behaviors of laboratory animals. Increasing levels of the arousal-related transmitter can elevate the expression of aggressive behaviors, while decreasing levels can reduce offensive aggression (pp. 126–7). Likewise, increasing levels of norepinephrine in the synapse by blocking release of norepinephrine from the synapse "increased aggressive behavior of isolated mice confronting each other." Genetic manipulations which have the effect of increasing norepinephrine lead to mice that show higher levels of aggressive behavior.

What about dopamine as an arousal-related transmitter? Miczek concludes that "aggressive behavior depends on intact dopamine neurons in the mesocorticolimbic pathways" (p. 127). Data focus on the role of dopamine in initiating aggression.

"Destroying these dopaminergic systems with a specific neurotoxin, 6-OHDA decreases offensive aggression and exaggerates defensive ragelike reactions" (p. 127). To follow-up Miczek's work, my lab studied gene dosage effects, dealing with the gene for catechol-O-methyltransferase, coding for an enzyme important in the chemical break-down of norepinephrine and dopamine (Gogos et al., 1998). Interestingly, heterozygotes for this gene's knockout showed strikingly lower latencies for aggressive behavior and, cor-respondingly, strikingly higher frequencies of aggression. But this is really a gene dos-age phenomenon because homozygous gene knockouts did not show these phenomena. I interpret the heterogyous knockout effect as being due to the fact that a decreased rate of breakdown of dopamine and norepinephrine would cause higher levels of these arousal-related transmitters in synapses. Clearly, dopamine working through dopamine type-2 receptors in the anterior hypothalamus contributes to aggressive behavior (reviewed, Melloni and Ricci, 2010). Further, mice bearing a knockout of the dopamine transporter gene – resulting in more dopamine in the synapse – are more likely to attack. For another example, the excitatory neurotransmitter glutamate stimulates aggression (reviewed, Melloni and Ricci, 2010). The inhibitory transmitter GABA presents a more complex situ-ation, but when it does inhibit aggression it does so through the GABA-A receptor.

Glutamate is a uniformly excitatory neurotransmitter. Miczek proposes that "one function of glutamate may be to exaggerate the excitability of neural systems responsible for aggressive behavior, particularly when aggression is intense" (p. 130). This interpreta-tion fits perfectly with the idea that aggression comprises a class of behaviors associated with high GA. The kind of data Miczek cites include the demonstration that a glutamate receptor subtype agonist's administration into an arousal-related brain region, the mid-brain periaqueductal gray, decreases the threshold there for electrical stimulation of a "defensive rage" pattern of aggressive behavior. That said, the differing affinities of various drugs for glutamate receptor subtypes as well as the phenomenon of receptor desensitiza-tion make for a complex literature. Overall, the behavioral results with various manipula-tions of neurotransmitter chemistry indicate that high levels of GA permit more frequent or intense aggressive behavior by experimental animals.

Daniel Pine, at the National Institute for Mental Health, discusses aggression in chil-dren (Blair et al., 2006). Hypervigilance, a heightened state of alertness of threat, well described in animal behavior, characterizes the behavior of children who are prone to reac-tive aggression. In addition, he notes that children with the high levels of arousal in anxious states are also prone to reactive aggression and other forms of anti-social behavior (p. 356).

Drugs of abuse often give sets of contradictory and confusing results with respect to the regulation of aggression due to the differing effects of different doses, as well as the effects of environmental context (Grimes and Melloni, p. 371 in Nelson, 2006). In contrast, diazepam administration to experimental animals, positively modifying GABA receptors, produces a widely recognized result: the reduction of aggression. This is true for a range of doses and for mice experienced with exposures to aggression, for isolation-induced aggression, and for other testing paradigms. Wall, Blanchard, and Blanchard (in Mattson, 2003) also cover pharmacologic effects on aggression. A main finding is that benzodiazepine agonists, anxiolytics (again working through GABA receptors), reduce defensive behaviors and attach behaviors in laboratory rats and mice. Complexities in this literature include occasional surprising findings with extremely low doses, distinc-tions between different kinds of aggression, and indirect effects. In this case, reduction of GA is associated with reduction of aggression.

Regarding the psychopharmacology of human aggression, Don Cherek describes studies in which regular cocaine users had increased incidence of violent behavior. On the other hand, he also quotes studies with benzodiazepines which reported increased aggressive responses. Therefore, even though some of the results with human subjects fit the idea of higher GA predisposing to aggression, findings were not uniform in that respect.

A broader view is taken by Fordham University Law Professor Deborah Denno (1990), interested in the full range of biological and environmental influences on violence and criminality. With respect to GA, she draws a connection to hyperactivity (p. 15) which, however, affects a heterogeneous group of children. Additional factors included maternal educational level, early disciplinary problems, and other problems involving familial instability.

In general, quoting Cal Tech Professor David Anderson (2016), CNS "arousal effects apply to humans and animals and involve increases in physiological autonomic and motor activities and increased sensitivity to sensory cues. They increase the probability of engaging in aggression."

Interoception. For all three parts of this chapter, the concept of "interoception" is important. The great American psychologist William James, in the James-Lange theory of emotion, argued that interoception, the perceptions of physiological changes in our bodies, are essential for the experience of emotion. As Lisa Feldman Barrett reminds us (2017), the ascending signals from autonomic system neurons that serve interoception inform the brain about the state of our viscera (all the organs and tissues inside the trunk of our body), muscles, joints, temperature, energy level, etc. Thus, one set of factors contributing to high levels of GA comprise those interoceptive, autonomic nervous system signals informing the brainstem that, in fact, our bodies are ready for high levels of GA.

Classically, neuroscientists have understood that autonomic system neurons, both sympathetic (e.g., higher heart rate, higher blood pressure) and parasympathetic (vasodilation, gastrointestinal motility), participate in emotion and arousal. As well, these neurons signal the states of our viscera to the brain (Levenson, 2003). Some of the autonomically mediated physiological changes are visible, such as the reddening of the skin and constriction of the pupils during anger and the blanching of the skin and dilation of the pupils during fear. Azevedo et al. (2017) investigated the role of GA as a determinant of emotional experience, not just a consequence of that experience. They reported an effect of heart rate phase on attention to images of fearful faces. They found "selective enhancement of attentional engagement to low spatial frequency fearful faces presented during the cardiac systole (high blood pressure) relative to diasole" (low blood pressure). Even more startling with respect to the role of the autonomic nervous system in GA as required for consciousness, a group of French neurologists (Corazzol et al., Current Biology, 2017) recently reported that long-term stimulation of the vagus nerve of a patient who was in a vegetative state for 15 years heightened GA "sustained attention, body motility and visual pursuit. Scores on the Coma Recovery Scale-Revised (CRS-R) test improved, mostly in the visual domain, as stimulation increased, from a score of 5 at baseline (last exam) to 10 at highest intensities (1.00–1.25 mA), indicating a transition from a vegetative to minimally conscious state." In similar work, Heesink et al. (2017) tested military veterans with anger and aggression problems on measures of startle responses and compared their results to veteran "controls" who had no such problems. The veterans with anger problems had increased electromyographic responses to the startling stimuli, and the result was consistent with personality analyses called "State Anger and Harm Avoidance." These veterans must have had higher levels of GA in order to give strong and rapid responses. The authors concluded that "threat reactivity is increased in anger and aggression problems." It appears that autonomic system neurons participate in supporting GA as well as the physiological aspects of emotion.

A recent and very surprising report by Alvarez-Dieppa, working with C. K. McIntyre at the University of Texas (2016) indicates that vagus nerve stimulation (VNS) enhances the consolidation of extinction of conditioned fear. Freezing, as a fear response, was significantly reduced in VNS-extinction rats. Again, a link from a part of the autonomic system to a high GA behavior.

Thus for all three types of behaviors considered in this chapter – aggression, fear, and sex – signals from the autonomic nervous systems that they are active, in a way that would support GA, constitutes one way in which GA participates in these three classes of high-arousal behaviors.

Androgenic Hormones, Testosterone. High levels of testosterone in the blood facilitate aggression in experimental animals and in men; they also heighten arousal. Some medical doctors claim that giving testosterone to older males makes them more energetic, alert, excitable, and happy. I will instead concentrate on controlled laboratory tests which focus on physiological variables such as blood pressure, and behavioural variables such as alertness, attention, and mood. The neuroscience laboratory of Elliott Albers at Georgia State led the way in showing that testosterone effects on specific groups of neurons in the basal forebrain encourage aggression in male laboratory animals (Albers, 2015; Caldwell and Albers, 2016). For example, he pinpointed neurons that express the neuropeptide vasopressin as important for androgenic stimulation of male aggression. Accordingly, when male laboratory animals are castrated, vasopressin levels are markedly reduced, and so is aggression. Put briefly, testosterone raises activity in neurons that promote aggression and reduces activity in neurons that inhibit aggression. Testosterone's most obvious route of action would be through its facilitation of the expression of specific genes in the brain (Figure 7.1).

Harrison Pope, at Harvard Medical School, was the first scientist to draw testosterone directly into causation of human aggression. But if you reflect for a moment on the hyper-muscular roles in various dramas or the real-life phenomenon of "'roid rage," the scientific proof could be considered obvious. Pope's work complements a huge set of studies on human aggressive behaviors summarized in Randy Nelson's *Biology of Aggression.*

With respect to testosterone, what about physiological components of aggression that depend on high GA? Rasmussen et al. (2017) found that users of androgenic steroids had higher systolic blood pressure than controls. Conversely, in rats with normal blood pressure and in a strain of rats with spontaneous hypertension, castration to reduce testosterone levels also caused mean arterial pressure to decrease (Loh and Salleh, 2017). In a molecular pharmacological study, Dordea et al. (2016) uncovered a "testosterone-dependent impairment of acetylcholine-induced relaxation," meaning that testosterone obliterated one mechanism for lowering blood pressure. High salt in the diet is accompanied by high blood pressure, and castration prevents that elevation (Oloyo et al., 2016). Iams and Wexler (1979) studied young male rats that become spontaneously hypertensive when they mature. Castration "retarded the usual steep ascent of blood pressure." In summary, several studies show that higher levels of testosterone cause the higher blood pressure which accompanies high GA behaviors.

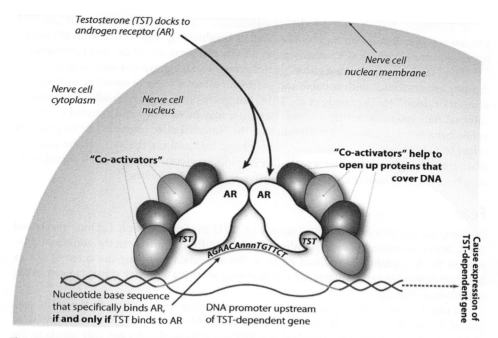

Figure 7.1 Effect of testosterone (TST) on DNA transcription in TST-susceptible neurons. TST enters the nucleus from the neuronal cytoplasm after binding to the androgen receptor (AR). Only when TST is bound to the AR do the co-activator proteins that cover the coiled DNA open up the chromatin, uncovering and uncoiling the DNA to allow gene transcription. Uncoiling enables the TST-carrying AR to interact with the DNA nucleotide base sequence of the promoter that commands the downstream expression of TST-dependent genes ("downstream" is off the right side of the diagram). I propose that differences among individuals in their co-activator chemistry likely account for some of the differences among young men in their propensities toward aggression (From Pfaff et al., 2011)

What about behavioral measures? Fontani et al. (2004) reported that higher levels of testosterone were significantly correlated with high levels of alertness. In experimental animals, Archer (1977) built on studies showing that testosterone increases persistence of food searching in chicks, and found the same phenomenon in mice. Likewise, males with normal testosterone levels males investigated novel conspecifics significantly longer than castrates investigated (Thor et al., 1982). With respect to information processing by humans, Chen et al. (2015) reported that testosterone is capable of heightening alertness such that during tests of vocal threat processing, testosterone shortened latencies of response.

Mood changes have also been examined. Wang et al. (1996) studied the effect of testosterone replacement on changes in mood; it was studied for 60 days in 51 hypogonadal men. When compared with a control, baseline period, testosterone replacement led to significant decreases in anger, irritability, and sadness. With testosterone, there was a significant improvement in energy level, friendliness, and sense of well-being. Wang concluded that testosterone replacement therapy in hypogonadal men improved their positive mood parameters, such as energy, well/good feelings, and friendliness; it decreased negative mood parameters including anger, nervousness, and irritability.

In summary, testosterone heightens autonomic reactivity, alertness, attention, and persistence that depend on high GA, as well as heightening aggression. And, of course, aggression requires high GA, autonomic reactivity alertness, attention, and persistence.

David Anderson (2016) asks how "goal-directed social behaviours such as mating and fighting are associated with scalable and persistent internal states of emotion, motivation, arousal or drive." He (Kennedy et al., 2014) "suggests possible ways in which changes in internal state intensity during a social encounter may be encoded and coupled to appropriate behavioral decisions." I maintain that the "internal state intensity" he emphasizes refers to GA, required for aggression (above) and fear and sex (below). By the way, if a scale-free GA network facilitates scale-free (rapidly accelerating) behavior, it would facilitate both rapid-offensive and rapid-defensive aggressive behaviors.

Fear

Building on the pioneering contributions of NYU Professor Joseph LeDoux (reviewed 2000, 2014), we begin by understanding clearly that direct paths from the auditory thalamus to the amygdala and indirect paths to the amygdala involving the cerebral cortex both participate in mechanisms for fear learning when an auditory signal is used as the conditional stimulus.

In order to relate the large body of data concerning fear learning to the main subject of this book, I must refer to the work of James McGaugh's lab, at the University of California, Irvine. Benno Roozendaal and McGaugh showed years ago that inputs to the amygdala from brainstem arousal systems are necessary for efficient fear learning performance (Roozendaal et al 1999) (Figure 7.2). McGaugh's lab (LaLumiere et al., 2017) has recently reviewed how emotional arousal during the learning consolidation period influences and enhances the strength of the fear memory. "Emotional arousal activates systems that influence" how fear memories are processed, "specifically leading to enhanced memory consolidation compared with memories for emotionally neutral or mundane events. In addition, emotionally arousing events may also activate the basolateral amygdala through other means."

Consistent with the emphasis in the McGaugh lab's data about arousal transmitter effects in the amygdala, Schwabe et al. (2013) found *blocking* an adrenoreceptor reduced the subsequent memory for emotional pictures. In my lab, studies with mice bearing a knockout of a gene whose product is an enzyme important for the breakdown of norepinephrine and dopamine also yielded a sex-specific result (Gogos et al., 1998). Females bearing the knockout showed high anxiety-like behavior: long latencies to emerge from the dark chamber into the lighted part and less time walking around in the light. Males did not show that result.

Neuroanatomy. I am convinced that our feeling of fear depends on the electrical activity of neurons in the human amygdala. Long ago, neuroanatomists thought of the amygdala as a single structure, named because when viewed in the human brain from below, it is shaped like an almond (the Greek name for almond is "amygdala"). Now we know that the amygdala has more than 10 subdivisions which have different roles. Rather than delving into all of those, we'll take a straightforward three-step approach to explaining fear: (i) How do danger signals get to the amygdala? (ii) How do fear messages radiate out from the amygdala? (iii) What are the nerve cells in the amygdala doing to execute that transformation from input to output?

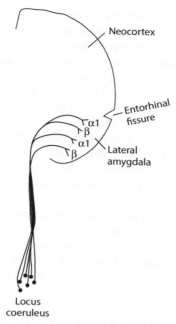

Neocortex

Entorhinal
fissure

α1
β
α1
β

Lateral
amygdala

Locus
coeruleus

Figure 7.2 Data from the laboratory of Professor James McGaugh (references in text) and others show the importance, for fear learning, of arousal-promoting noradrenergic (norepinephrine) inputs to the amygdala

First, sensory signals which warn us of danger converge on the amygdala using a variety of routes. We mainly divide them up according to whether they go through the thalamus (which is also the path for signals destined for the cerebral cortex), or whether they avoid the thalamus. The latter, non-thalamic signals, come both from the classical olfactory system that handles an infinite variety of different smells, and from the more specialized accessory olfactory system which handles pheromones, among other odors. Thalamic neurons signal all the other danger signs: visual, auditory, taste, and touch. In modern neurobiology, the auditory warnings of danger are the best-known because NYU Professor Joseph LeDoux (2000, 2014) has been so successful at analyzing exactly how they work. As noted, LeDoux has shown how a sound that warns the animal of a painful foot shock can use projections directly from thalamus to amygdala, or a less direct route which loops into the cortex on the way to the amygdala. He characterizes the direct path as faster and the cortical mechanism as more accurate. Both enter the amygdala in its lateral subdivision. In the lateral amygdala, in addition to excitatory transmission related to fear, GABA-mediated signaling plays a complex role (Liu et al., 2017). GABA-A synapses inhibit electrical activity as expected, but when the delta subunit-containing is present, disinhibition of activity actually facilitates the expression of fear. The authors think of this result as "tuning" the inhibitory tone in the lateral amygdala thus to "prevent excessive suppression" and ensure that fear can be expressed when necessary.

Secondly, when the amygdala has done its job, what happens? Amygdaloid messages radiate widely in the brain, including the frontal cortex, the hypothalamus, and the midbrain, accomplishing a variety of tasks that we associate with fear. Axons going to the hypothalamus can activate our autonomic nervous systems – blood pressure, heart rate, sweating, and so forth – and can influence hormonal outputs from the pituitary gland that dangles from the bottom of the hypothalamus. The hormonal changes can be fast, because the tiny nine-amino-acid vasopressin can protect us from blood loss if we are wounded. Or they can be slow, since the large protein hormone adrenocortical trophic hormone, ACTH, will turn on the adrenal gland so as to release stress hormones. Some amygdaloid axons take a long route all the way down to the midbrain. There neurons found absolutely in the middle of the midbrain, the central gray, cause the immediate reflex response to fear. A laboratory animal anticipating painful shock will freeze immediately, sometimes for quite a long time, before taking the next step. Additionally, what about the obvious intellectual or psychological components of fear? Amygdaloid axons going to our cerebral cortex should contribute to an explanation of how frightening events are registered in human emotion.

Third, between inputs and outputs of the amygdala, nerve cells with extremely short axons are getting the job done within the amygdala itself. Best established is the axonal projection from the lateral region of the amygdala into the central region (the "central nucleus"). David J. Anderson has used the most modern genetic and molecular techniques to piece together a story about how neurons within the amygdala manage to activate fear. Anderson focused on the different kinds of neurons in the central nucleus, some on its lateral and some on its medial side. Most importantly, he used very brief light pulses and specialized viruses to solve a major problem in contemporary neurobiology: when different kinds of neurons are next to each other, how do you influence one kind without at the same time influencing the other? First, Anderson's lab members identified a chemical constituent of inhibitory neurons, so-called PKC-delta, on the lateral side of the central nucleus. Then they used their knowledge of the PKC-delta gene to create a neuroanatomical marker and to show that those neurons send axons over to the medial side of the central nucleus. Those axons would be thought to inhibit the medial neurons. Finally, after electrical recording experiments to verify their methodology, they suppressed neuronal activity in these PKC-delta neurons and caused elevated levels of fear. They concluded that the lateral side of the central nucleus contains an "inhibitory microcircuit" that in turn regulates an inhibitory connection over to the medial neurons (Haubensak et al., 2010). Knock down that latter inhibition, and fear increases.

Anderson also has ventured outside the amygdala to investigate another part of the limbic system, the lateral septum. The lateral septum receives inputs from the amygdala. Todd Anthony, working with Anderson, modified a particular set of lateral septum neurons that express a special receptor for CRF, mentioned above. Once modified, these neurons could be activated by brief light pulses sent into the septum even when other neurons nearby would not be activated. The bottom line is that activating these CRF-receiving neurons in the septum increased anxiety-like behaviors when mice were stressed. Thus, the amygdala and its outputs, with an emphasis on the neuropeptide CRF, tell us how, in neuroanatomical and neurochemical terms, fear and stress feed into an anxious disposition.

Anderson and his team have pieced together a neurobiological story that most scientists can only dream of. They have related expression of specific genes in identified neurons of a mammalian brain to the causes of a global behavioral state.

One complexity of fear learning concerns the choice between active and passive fear responses. Fadok et al. (2017) noted that in the face of threat, animals may freeze, a passive response, but they may also make an escape response, active flight. These authors used optogenetic techniques to show that different neurons in the central nucleus of the amygdala regulate passive versus active fear responses. The two sets of amygdaloid neurons are mutually inhibitory. Nerve cells expressing corticotrophic releasing hormone (CRH) mediate active flight responses, while somatostatin-expressing neurons are responsible for freezing.

Hormones. This recent CRH discovery echoed previous work. Louis Muglia is a molecular endocrinologist and a pediatrician. Working with his team, then at Washington University in Saint Louis, he brought two hormones associated with stress and fear into relation with the amygdaloid neuronal mechanisms just mentioned (Kolber et al., 2008). Cortisol (in animals, corticosterone) is a steroid hormone exquisitely responsive to stress and fear. It regulates gene expression in cells with its receptors in their cell nuclei, including cells in the amygdala. One of the neurochemicals it regulates is abbreviated CRF (or CRH), which, like a tiny protein called a neuropeptide, has two separate roles: CRF directs the pituitary gland to send hormonal signals to the adrenal glands, thus to produce more cortisol; crucially, CRF acts in the brain itself to direct the organism's responses to fear and stress. In a clever series of experiments, Muglia and his team used viral vectors to knock out expression of cortisol's nuclear receptor in the central nucleus of the amygdala. The mice which received this treatment showed much less conditioned fear. Putting CRF back into the brain of such mice restored fear behavior. Muglia's team concluded that fear required cortisol signaling in the central nucleus of the amygdala with the consequence of CRF signaling and, thence, fear.

While the most discriminating analyses of amygdala neurons have been carried out in laboratory animals, I am convinced that the conclusions of such analyses apply to the human brain. For example, as noted above, Leslie Ungerleider (Pessoa and Ungerleider, 2004; Hadj-Bouziane et al., 2012), at the National institute of Mental Health, and Ralph Adolphs, at Cal Tech, have shown the importance of the human amygdala for modulating behavioral responses to different types of faces (Harrison et al., 2015; Wang et al., 2017). Kerry Ressler's lab (Stevens et al., 2017) at Emory University and Harvard have recently used functional magnetic resonance imaging (fMRI) to study patients from a trauma center and report "neural signatures of risk for maintaining post-traumatic stress disorder symptoms: amygdala reactivity and habituation in the anterior cingulated cortex both correlated with the unfortunate maintenance of symptoms twelve months after trauma." All of these studies with human subjects illustrate how a well-developed field of research with laboratory animals can evolve into a field of work with importance for humans.

The level of molecular detail approached by current studies is illustrated by a microRNA analysis of the basolateral amygdala. Murphy et al. (2017) used mice in which fear extinction was impaired, and found that dietary tricks used to improve extinction were accompanied by changes in the levels of microRNAs in the amygdala. One candidate, miR-144-3p, was perfectly correlated with behavioral changes. Overexpression of this microRNA in the basolateral amygdala not only improved fear extinction but also protected against fear renewal. Now the known targets of this microRNA will come under vigorous study.

Even though the studies cited here show how amygdala neurons and circuits can participate in the regulation of fear, their activity does not simply stand in as the *only* neurophysiological representation of fear. It is not true that under all circumstances amygdaloid circuits are necessary and sufficient for fear. Lisa Feldman Barrett (2017) points out examples in which people with damaged amygdalae can feel fear. Also, there is a developmental disability, the Urbach-Wiethe disease, in which parts of the amygdalae are absent but, as Barrett describes, "other networks are compensating for (the patient's) missing amygdalae," when the patient shows normal fear responses (pp. 18–19).

Along this line of thought, some of the connections between GA and fear learning take place long after the original fear conditioning. At MIT, the laboratory of Susumu Tonegawa (Kitamura et al., 2017) concluded that the memory of the painful shock depended at first on hippocampal neurons whose activity "became silent with time," whereas prefrontal cortex neurons whose memory of the fear became functionally mature with time (more than 11 days). Likewise, Marin et al. (2017), studying (delayed) fear extinction in patients with anxiety disorders (compared to controls), found significantly less activation in the prefrontal cortex of the patients. Thus, later in the temporal sequence of a high GA event – be it painful shock in animals or high anxiety in patients – the prefrontal cortex comes into play.

More about Arousal. Fear learning expert Gregory Quirk (2016) portrays fear as "a bodily response to threat" and fear responses as a "set of behavioral, autonomic, and hormonal responses," all requiring high levels of arousal. The day I wrote this paragraph newspapers reported the mass shooting in Las Vegas, and I could imagine the panic of the crowd being shot at, all in hyper-arousal. As noted above and as reviewed by Joseph LeDoux (2000, 2014), the amygdala constitutes a crucial set of neuronal cell groups for fear conditioning. The importance of the amygdala has been shown by experiments in several species. For example, if the conditioned stimulus for a painful shock is auditory, inputs to the lateral subnucleus of the amygdala from the auditory thalamus, the auditory cortex, and the midbrain's periaqueductal gray (for GA) are involved. As noted when referring to David Anderson's work, the key connection inside the amygdala is from the lateral to the central subnucleus. From the central amygdala emanates a wide range of outputs to the hypothalamus and brainstem, including those which speak of high GA: the lateral hypothalamus (higher heart rate, sweaty skin, blood pressure elevation, pupil dilation), the parabrachial nucleus (panting), the locus coeruleus, and the lower brainstem reticular formation (increased startle response). Within amygdala neurons, molecular mechanisms involved include "a calcium/calmodulin-dependent kinase cascade, a protein kinase family of enzymes and tyrosine kinase pathways" (Quirk, 2016, p. 2420).

In summary, almost 50 years of neuroscientific research on brain mechanisms underlying fear attest to the importance of arousal-related neurotransmitters and hormones in fear and fear learning. Moreover, it is fair to say that in response to a dire threat, it is not just "part of the brain" that reacts in fear. It is the entire brain. Therefore, the A/P, L generalized arousal system serves well. Long distance connections spewing out identical, well-integrated signals are perfectly appropriate for initiating fearful behavior and escape.

Sex

Brain mechanisms for both female and male reproductive behaviors have been studied intensively in laboratory animals. They obviously have close relations with mechanisms of GA.

Female. The primary female mating behavior depends on estrogenic hormones acting through estrogen receptor-alpha in neurons of the ventromedial nucleus of the hypothalamus. Outputs from these neurons reach the midbrain central gray, where they activate a spinal–brainstem–spinal circuit sufficient for executing the behavior. Estrogen receptor-alpha is a ligand-activated transcription factor, and over the years we discovered several genes which have two properties: estrogens raise their mRNA concentrations in hypothalamus, and their gene products foster female reproductive behavior (reviewed in Pfaff, 2017).

Arousal. Female rodent mating behaviors obviously depend on high GA. First, the behaviors themselves. They involve rapid locomotion, sudden stops, and the need to support the weight of the mounting male (Pfaff, 1980; Garey et al., 2002). All of these speak of high GA. Further, high arousal resulting from olfactory inputs processed via the vomeronasal organ and accessory olfactory bulb seems to be essential for the expression of lordosis in hormone-primed female subjects (McCarthy et al., 2017).

Female mating behaviors depend on arousal-related neurotransmitters acting on hypothalamic neurons (reviewed, Pfaff, 2017). Further, the work of University of Maryland Professor Jessica Mong knowing that "methamphetamine is a psychomotor stimulant strongly associated with increases in sexual drive and behavior in women and men", Holder and Mong (2010) used female rats to show that repeated exposure to METH enhances both sexual receptivity and courtship behaviors. Then (2015) they examined the mechanisms underlying the drug–sex interaction. "Infusion of a Dopamine type-1 receptor agonist into the medial amygdala increased proceptive (courtship) behavior, while infusion of a D1 receptor antagonist blocked the ability of METH to increase proceptive behaviors." In 2017, using a technique for neuronal inactivation, they further reported that the ovarian steroid/methamphetamine responsive cells in the medial amygdala are necessary for meth-induced facilitation of proceptive behaviors. All of this pharmacological evidence connects female reproductive behavior to high GA.

Estrogenic effects on sexual arousal are not unique, in that estrogens also heighten several other aspects and manifestations of behavioral arousal: pain locomotion, aggression, anxiety, and the sleep–wake cycle. We deal with these five aspects, in order: (i) Estrogens can increase pain sensitivity (Dina et al., 2001; LaCroix-Fralish et al., 2005; Hucho et al., 2006; Claiborne et al., 2009) working through estrogen receptor-alpha (even as they decrease pain sensitivity through ER-beta). (ii) Clearly, estrogens elevate arousal as measured by the initiation of locomotor activity, acting through ER-alpha (Ogawa et al., 2003), perhaps because they lower adenosine 2A receptor gene expression in the ventrolateral preoptic area (Ribeiro et al., 2009). In fact, viral vector-mediated overexpression of ER-alpha in the striatum increases estradiol-induced motor activity (Schultz et al., 2009). (iii) New results suggest that even as the long-term effects of estrogens on aggression through ER-alpha depend on the sex of the animal studied (Ogawa et al., 2004), acute activation of ER-beta increases specific aspects of aggressive behaviors in mice, namely, those aggressive responses that are not directly involved in attacks. (iv) Estrogenic effects on anxiety and fear are complex, and appear to depend both upon the assay used and on the ER subtype through which estrogens are operating (Lunga and Herbert, 2004; Lund et al., 2005; Hiroi and Neumaier, 2006). (v) Finally, in laboratory animals, estrogens are associated with decreases in slow-wave sleep (Li and Satinoff, 1996; Colvin et al., 1969; Colvin et al., 1968), perhaps because of the ability of estrogens to suppress the activity of neurons in a sleep-producing neuronal group, the ventrolateral preoptic area (Mong et al., 2003a, b; Peterfi et al., 2004; Hadjimarkou et al., 2008; Devidze et al., 2010). Neurochemically, it has been shown that estrogens and orexin interact in their effects on measures of arousal in female mice (Easton et al., 2006). In women, under

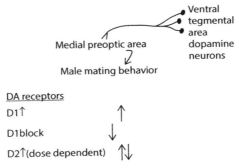

Figure 7.3 Based upon reviews by Professor Elaine Hull (2017), one sees that effects of the arousal-promoting neurotransmitter dopamine (DA) on male mating behavior are dose-dependent

certain conditions, estrogens clearly heighten mood (Gillies and McArthur, 2010; Maki et al., 2010; Ng et al., 2010; Sundermann et al., 2010) and "increase blood perfusion of cortical areas involved in cognitive tasks" (Dietrich et al., 2001).

Males. Male reproductive behavior depends on the actions of either testosterone or estrogens on neurons in the medial preoptic area (just in front of the hypothalamus) (reviewed by Hull, 2016). Inputs from olfactory and pheromonal signals to the preoptic area are important. Outputs from the medial preoptic area travel posteriorly through the lateral hypothalamus to reach the midbrain. Male behaviors in these laboratory animals being more complicated than female behaviors, the circuitry becomes obscure downstream from the midbrain.

Arousal. Testosterone effects on arousal-related behaviors and on autonomic arousal were covered above. But what about male laboratory animals which have normal testosterone levels but are still sluggish, not mating. It is well known that a GA-heightening tail pinch will stimulate mating performance. Likewise, a flank skin electrical shock, to heighten GA, stimulated precocious mating in male rats (Goldfoot and Baum, 1972). Finally, a very recent paper showed that optogenetic activation of arousing pheromonal-signaling (accessory olfactory bulb) mitral cell inputs (probably to the medial amygdala) augmented mating performance in male mice (Kunkhyen et al., 2017).

Further, arousal-related transmitters such as dopamine are important (Figure 7.3).

We sought to determine, by breeding lines of mice for high or low generalized arousal (GA), whether genetically encoded differences in generalized arousal would translate into alterations in specific types of arousal-dependent motivated behaviors. To that end, we took the mice of generation number 7, in the breeding project, and divided them in two different ways, by (1) parental arousal – whether their parents were in the high or low lines and (2) offspring arousal – whether the animal in question (G6) was at the top or bottom of the arousal distribution (Weil et al., 2010). First, male mice were exposed to a sexually naïve conspecific (of the Het8 strain) on consecutive days until they mated. Males from the high line and those offspring who exhibited high levels of GA exhibited a specific pattern of sexual behavior associated with a higher level of excitability and sexual arousal. High arousal males exhibited more mounts before intromission, and, then, fewer intromissions before ejaculating, and they ejaculated more quickly after the first intromission. Additionally, the percentage of mount attempts that were successful in leading to intromission was significantly lower among male mice from the high arousal line. The pattern of sexual behavior indicates that high-arousal males were highly excitable in an inappropriate manner, as indicated by the very low intromission–total mount ratio. The low arousal males showed patterns of sexual behavior exactly opposite to high-arousal. Thus, breeding males for high or low generalized CNS arousal produced animals whose sexual arousal was high or low, respectively (Weil et al., 2010).

Summary

It is clear from a variety of genetic, pharmacological, and biophysical studies that heightened generalized CNS arousal can foster increased sexual arousal, and the reverse (reviewed, Schober et al., 2011). Therefore, the prediction from generalized arousal theory is satisfied, that its perturbations should be able to alter specific, motivated behaviors.

Further, the universality of GA systems among vertebrates match the universality of sexual, fearful, and aggressive behaviors for which high GA is required.

8 Phase Transitions from Low GA States

Not all useful mental processes are conscious. Consider implicit learning (which we do without realizing it), implicit memory (recall without realizing that we know something), and embodied cognition ("mental functioning based on our body") (Weinberger, 2018). Nobel laureate Daniel Kahneman and Amos Tversky (2011) wrote about unconscious cognitive strategies, and Sigmund Freud's psychoanalytic theories posited unconscious emotions and motivations.

So, unconscious processes exist, but the purpose of this chapter is to explore mechanisms by which our brains emerge from the states of lowest GA, deep anesthesia, deep sleep, and traumatic brain injury. Here I relate modern neuroscience's understanding of mechanisms involved in the brain's recovery – toward and into consciousness – from deep anesthesia, deep sleep, and traumatic brain injury. Comparisons among these three states of low GA are inherently difficult, but below this chapter quotes the best paper dealing with the comparison (Brown et al., 2010).

Anesthesia

In keeping with the book's title, I am exploring the mechanisms which are effective in promoting the transition from unconsciousness to the lower states of awareness. For example, Chapter 2 introduced data from Rockefeller lab leader, neurophysiologist Diany Paola Calderon, that manipulating NGC neurons could alter the state of anesthesia of the cortex (Calderon et al., 2018; see Figure 8.1).

If anesthesia uses particular mechanisms, then, some of the paths toward consciousness likely use the reverse. Thus, understanding anesthesia reveals insights about the reverse, i.e., paths toward consciousness. Writing in the Hemmings and Hopkins (2006) text, Columbia professor Neil Harrison (p. 288 ff) identifies molecular targets of anesthetics. It is clear that anesthetics have important effects at both pre- and post-synaptic sites. One common example is the ability of isoflurane to enhance GABA-a receptor function. Isoflurane can also activate potassium "leak" channels which would serve to hyperpolarize neurons and lower their activity. Barbiturates also allosterically modulate GABA-a receptors in such a way as to potentiate inhibitory actions. The result (O'Pryor and Veselis, p. 349ff) is a loss of consciousness.

Detailed biophysical studies of the anesthetic process (Herold et al., 2017) yield surprising results. A new technique called a gramicidin channel measures direct effects on membrane lipids. Membrane lipid properties were only affected at anesthetic doses higher than that routinely used during surgery, leading to the inference that that "anesthetics directly interact with membrane proteins without altering lipid bilayer mechanical properties at clinically relevant concentrations."

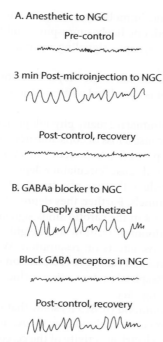

Figure 8.1 A simple cartoon of neurophysiologist Paola Calderon's results showing that an anesthetic (isoflurane) microinjected exclusively into Nucleus GigantoCellularis (NGC) can reduce cortical arousal, and that deep anesthesia can be partly blocked by opposing NGC inhibition. (A) Under conditions where the cortical electroencephalogram (EEG) was activated (low amplitude, high frequency wave activity), microinjection of anesthetic directly to NGC caused a sleep-typical EEG (high amplitude, low frequency). (B) The anesthetic is known to use inhibitory GABA synapses. Blocking GABA-a receptors specifically in NGC changed the EEG from high amplitude, low frequency waves to an activated condition (low amplitude, high frequency waves) (Calderon et al., 2018)

Which membrane proteins interact with anesthetics? Voltage-gated sodium channels. Anesthetics inhibit channel function "by reducing peak Na^+ current and shifting steady-state inactivation toward more hyperpolarized potentials" (Herold et al., 2017). Sand et al.'s (2017) biophysical model indicates that isoflurane modulates presynaptic sodium channel gating primarily by increasing forward activation and inactivation rate constants. These findings support accumulating evidence for "multiple sites of anesthetic interaction" with this sodium channel. In addition, at the 2017 meeting of the Society for Neuroscience Tamara Stamenic of the University of Colorado reported that a specific calcium channel, 3.1, acting in the central thalamus, is important for the ability of isoflurane to exert its usual action, increased slow-wave activity (delta) in the cortical electroencephalograph (EEG).

In terms of neuroanatomical sites of action, Donald Koblin (p. 109 ff. in Miller, 2005) emphasizes that while it is a commonly accepted notion that inhaled anesthetics work by decreasing activity in neurons of the brainstem reticular formation, effects on the forebrain are also likely important. However, decerebration (transection just behind the thalamus) does not alter anesthetic requirement. Koblin reasons that since successful anesthesia includes amnesia and immobility in response to pain, at least two different classes of sites must be involved: one likely supraspinal and the other spinal. In general, inhaled anesthetics that depress synaptic signaling are more effective than those affecting axonal conduction (p. 111).

A useful classical generalization called the Meyer-Overton rule states that higher lipid solubility of an anesthetic agent is correlated with anesthetic potency, but there are many exceptions.

Outside the brain we can summarize many physiological effects of anesthetics that by themselves are not thought to cause a loss of consciousness but which always accompany such loss (Pagel et al. in Miller, p. 191 ff). Anesthetics affect the heart. Virtually all of them "depress contractile function" and cause "circulatory depression," myocardial depression. This is in part because they reduce the size of a transient calcium flow and also affect L-type and T-type calcium channels. Further, they depress baroreceptor reflex control of blood pressure (stretch receptors in the carotid sinus signaling to the lower brainstem), and inhibit the sympathetic autonomic outflow that heightens blood pressure.

Additionally, anesthetics have effects on respiration. William Wilson and Jonathan Benumof (p. 679 ff) describe marked changes in respiration which differ according to the type and depth of anesthesia. Respiration depression includes decreased volumes, but the rate and smoothness of breathing vary.

Piyush Patel and John Drummond (p. 813 ff) show that virtually all anesthetics lower cerebral metabolic rate, but for cerebral blood flow the results vary across anesthetics.

What about changes in the electrical activity of the cerebral cortex itself? Mahla et al. (p. 1511 ff) describe the simplest changes in the electroencephalogram with the type of deep anesthesia dealt with in this chapter: increases in amplitude together with the loss of high frequencies (in the gamma and beta range, e.g., greater than 15 waves/second) and a descent into the lowest frequencies (e.g., delta range, 0.5 waves/second). Electrical potentials in the cortex evoked by sensory stimulation tend to become blunted (features of the complex potentials obscured) by deep anesthesia. There are exceptions to this general rule. For example, ketamine has little or no effect on evoked potentials.

While the classical EEG finding, dating back to the 1930s, is that there will be increased slow-wave activity during anesthesia, there are exceptions. For example, ketamine produces fast gamma oscillations, and the alpha-2 agonist dexmedetomidine produces sleep-like spindles.

Overall, it seems clear, from the work of Alex Proekt (Pennsylvania) and Emery Brown (Harvard) and others, that sophisticated mathematical analyses of EEG before and during surgery will make anesthesiology more precise than ever before.

Memory. Leading academic anesthesiologists are now concerned with the problems of memory and awareness in anesthesia (Kurata and Hemmings, 2015). It is not desirable for the patient to have intraoperative awareness of pain and procedures. Thus, doctors must attend to the difficult subject of the "subconscious processes of mind." Behavioral techniques and EEG analyses have not yet solved the problem. "No single reliable anaesthetic technique or monitor is yet available to eliminate awareness with recall." Understanding what happens during emergency is even harder. Andrew Hudson and Alex Proekt (see Hudson et al 2014) showed with mathematical statistical analyses that recovery of high-frequency EEG activity does *not* occur in the form of a simple monotonic curve which reflects decreasing anesthetic concentration in the brain. Rather, there are mathematically defined dwelling states, "hubs," which constitute dynamic way stations on the path from total unconsciousness to total consciousness. The actual, physiological network properties that correspond to these dwelling states remain to be identified.

Along these lines, Vazey and Aston-Jones (2014), knowing that mechanisms driving emergence from general anesthesia are not well understood surprised us by bringing the noradrenergic locus coeruleus (LC) into the conversation. They used virally delivered designer receptors to regulate activity of these norepinephrine (NE) neurons, to investigate their causal relationship with anesthetic state. Activation of these neurons produced cortical electroencephalograph activation under continuous deep isoflurane anesthesia. Importantly, it also "accelerated behavioral emergence from deep isoflurane anesthesia" which, in turn, could be pharmacologically reversed. Thus, noradrenergic neurotransmission can affect the emergence from isoflurane general anesthesia.

This subject, overall, is a concern, as considered by Kurata and Hemmings (2015), because, for obvious reasons, if the patient really can recall things that happened during surgery there can be important, negative psychological consequences for the patient.

Comparisons among Low GA states. Comparisons among the three lowest GA states – deep anesthesia, deep sleep, and brain trauma – are difficult because, by definition, the patient is not behaving, not telling you anything, whether you are a scientist or a clinician. The most comprehensive recent comparative treatment was offered by Emory Brown, Ralph Lydic, and Nicholas Schiff in the New England Journal of Medicine (2010), quoted here. The first and most obvious comparison has to do with the valences of these three low GA states according to normal human values. Humans want healthy sleep, do not want traumatic brain damage, and must rarely submit to deep anesthesia for surgery. Sleep is brain-managed, anesthesia is doctor-managed, and brain trauma is unmanaged.

During sleep, brain mechanisms cycle between two states – rapid eye movement (REM) sleep and non-REM sleep – at approximately 90-minute intervals, whereas coma due to brain injury is a state of profound unresponsiveness. Patients with severe disorders of consciousness may display the high-amplitude, low-frequency electroencephalic (EEG) activity seen in patients under general anesthesia. Emory Brown's most memorable statement, in my view, is that "general anesthesia is, in fact, a reversible drug-induced coma."

An interesting point of comparison features the details of emergence from each of the low GA states. If it occurs at all, emergence from low GA caused by traumatic brain injury is delayed, unpredictable, and supported by agonized families and heroic medical attention. Emergence from sleep is the opposite: rapid and predictable by recovery from sleep deprivation and time of day. As Brown et al. summarize: "Emergence from general anesthesia is a passive process that depends on the amounts of drugs administered; their sites of action, potency, and pharmacokinetics; the patient's physiological characteristics; and the type and duration of the surgery. Recovery from general anesthesia is generally assessed by monitoring physiological and behavioral signs. The return of spontaneous respirations is typically one of the first clinical signs observed once peripheral neuromuscular blockade is decreased. This marks the patient's return from a functional state that approximates brainstem death." As you would guess from the foregoing, heart rate and blood pressure typically increase. The anesthesiologist will look for "return of brain-stem reflexes to maintain spontaneous respirations and airway protection, even if there is no response to oral commands. The eyes may still not open spontaneously." As noted above, the recovery of electrical activity in the cerebral cortex is not a linear process and features mathematically defined "hubs" of distinct states that seem to be required

(Hudson and Proekt, 2014). Later the patient will pass through the minimally conscious state, and finally will be able to answer questions.

To emphasize, recovery from coma caused by traumatic brain injury may require years. In contrast, emergence from general anesthesia may require just minutes. Brown et al. make the interesting observation that "the early clinical signs of emergence from general anesthesia – return of regular breathing, salivation, tearing, swallowing, gagging, and grimacing – approximate the caudal–rostral progression in the brain stem of the return of sensory, motor, and autonomic function. A later sign, such as response to oral commands, indicates the return of cortical function."

As mentioned, the cortical EEG in sleep cycles through stages. The stage most *dissimilar* to anesthesia is REM sleep, which features a highly active cortex. Slow wave (deep, unresponsive) sleep is more similar to anesthesia, and is deep enough for surgery.

Ralph Lydic and Helen Baghdoyan, at the University of Michigan (Hemmings, Hopkins, p. 361 ff), contrast the drug-induced process of anesthetization with what they term physiologically generated sleep as an "active process." Thus, in their Table 30.1, they describe the *onset* of anesthesia as not altered by previous sleep or environmental factors, whereas sleep onset is influenced by both of those. In terms of *maintenance*, anesthesia depends on drug dose and can be held for very long times, while sleep depends on prior wakefulness and rotates through stages (see below). Regarding *offset*, full return from anesthetization can be slow, the rate being determined by anesthetic kinetics and metabolism, and unpleasant (e.g., nausea). Return from sleep is rapid and normally pleasant. Nothing about anesthesia depends on circadian rhythms, but sleep physiology is exquisitely circadian-influenced (see below).

Finally, leading cortical physiologist and consciousness theorist Christof Koch, now director of the Allen Institute for Brain Science, displays confidence (2017) in a new technique for measuring degrees of consciousness. In 2016, Sylvia Casaratto, of the University of Milan, and her team reported a method of using EEG, for estimating level of consciousness by charting the complex EEG responses to a sudden, single pulse of magnetic energy which emanates from a coil of wire held against the scalp. Such a measure might be useful, for example, with very young patients or with patients who are in variously reduced states of consciousness. Compressed, analyzed "complexity" of response correlated well when lined up with predictions (predictions from, for example, type and level of anesthetic). But some patients with disorders of consciousness displayed a much more complex EEG response than predicted. This highlights another major difference between anesthesia and traumatic brain injury (TBI). In anesthesia the loss of cerebral function is relatively uniform with a largely predictable distribution. In TBI, the injury and recovery patterns vary in time and space. In sum, manipulations of anesthetics provide one of the analytically cleanest approaches to the mechanisms and measurements of consciousness.

Sleep

According to a classical paper by Alexander Borbely (1982), well-regulated sleep depends on the time of day (read, "circadian rhythms") and the amount of time we have gone without sleep (homeostatic sleep need). I'll consider those two sets of mechanisms in order.

Circadian Rhythms. In 1971 Ronald Konopka, working in the laboratory of ex-physicist Seymour Benzer at California Institute of Technology (1971a, b), discovered three lines of mutant fruit flies in which circadian rhythms had been disrupted. One had too short a rhythm of locomotor activity (19 hours), one too long a rhythm (28 hours), and the third was totally arrhythmic. Konopka and Benzer surmised that all three mutants involved an individual gene on the X chromosome.

As genetic cloning techniques improved, the race was on to discover exactly what this gene is. Michael Young, working at Rockefeller University, reported in 1984 (Bargiello and Young, 1984) that they had isolated a single mRNA from the appropriate region of the X chromosome and they called the corresponding gene "period" as in the period of a rhythm (per). This transcript is eliminated by the Konopka/Benzer type of X chromosome mutation. Subsequent work (Saez and Young, 1988) localized per expression in cells in the eyes and optic lobes of the adult brain as well as other tissues. Leslie Vosshall et al. (1994) in the Young lab discovered a second clock gene "timeless" which regulates nuclear localization of PER and whose mutation also abolishes circadian rhythms. Vosshall and Young (1995) also found that expression of PER under the control of a promoter which is required for the development of fruit fly photoreceptors, in a few brain cells, is sufficient for behavioral rhythmicity.

Recently, Young has worked with physicist Eric Siggia (Kidd et al., 2015) to formulate and test a theory about the fruit fly rhythm's *in*sensitivity to environmental temperature. Their new theory posits that there exists "a gene circuit that responds only to temperature changes. This theory implies that temperature changes should linearly rescale the amplitudes of clock component oscillations but leave phase relationships and shapes unchanged." Data from TIMELESS expression measurements supported this prediction. Overall we are left with the current view (Top and Young, 2017) of several important clock genes in a complex and beautiful set of mechanisms. Gene products submit to regulated nuclear entry and regulated nuclear exit as they participate in more than 20 reactions. These reactions constitute the autoregulatory negative feedback relations which account for the clock's stability.

Meanwhile, in the Department of Biology at Brandeis University, Michael Rosbash and Jeffrey Hall were also on the trail of PER (reviewed, Hall and Rosbash, 1988). Their analyses (Reddy et al., 1984) agreed with Michael Young's and the combined effects of these labs' initiatives led to (a) a large and thriving field for the exploration of circadian mechanisms, (b) conclusions which apply to a wide variety of species, including mammals (Takahashi, 2016), and (c) a shared Nobel prize.

Neural and Metabolic Regulation. In the brain, the primary driving force to maintain a light-entrained circadian rhythm emanates from the suprachiasmatic nucleus of the hypothalamus (SCN). The history of work on the SCN was discussed in Chapter 5. In that chapter, it was impressive to see the several routes for circadian information to get from the SCN to other parts of the brain and body. In one such impressive demonstration, Gary Aston-Jones used trans-synaptic retrograde labeling to reveal several possible links from SCN to the LC (Aston-Jones et al., 2001). I emphasize that the manner in which SCN signals fan out through the brain provides the neural basis for widespread physiological effects. For example, Joseph Bass, from Northwestern, and Mitchell Lazar, at the University of Pennsylvania (2016), review how "circadian time signatures" are required for health. Glucose and fat metabolism in the liver, for example, insulin secretion by the pancreas, and the adrenal gland's stress hormone responses, among others, all must be timed right. If they are not, pathologies which correspond to each will break out (Bass and Lazar, 2016). As well, one can understand, in the words of Kevin Mann (2016), that "nearly every arm of the immune response (innate and adaptive) has been reported to oscillate in a circadian manner."

Neural network dynamics that regulate sleep have received much attention (Weber and Yan, 2016). Of special relevance, for this chapter, is Weber's review of neuronal groups whose activities promote the low GA state highlighted here, highlighting, for example, the brainstem nucleus of the solitary tract. A mathematical approach to network dynamics suggests that a set of 12 differential equations which express the activities of three coupled oscillators (representing sleep-active, REM-active, and wake-active neuronal populations) could simulate mouse sleep–wake timelines (Behn et al., 2007).

Physicist Marcelo Magnasco (Alonso et al., 2014; Solovey et al., 2015), at Rockefeller University, examined cortical electrical activity in humans using techniques with high temporal resolution. Their measurements revealed wave activity "at the boundary between stability and instability" leading to what Magnasco calls "dynamical criticality": a system poised to respond sensitively and rapidly to stimulus input. Magnasco's results support the theoretical proposal which physicist Jayanth Banavar and I put forward (Pfaff and Banavar, 2007), which drew the analogy between low GA/high GA transition and the physical phase transition displayed by liquid crystals. One concrete clue to this transition comes from my lab's recording of the human cortex's electrical activity during sleep. Human cortical arousals, displayed in the EEG, usually follow closely upon peripheral arousals, displayed in blood pressure measurements in the finger (Ribeiro et al., ms in preparation). A second route of experimentation in lab animals pits a motivational force like hunger against Borbely's circadian/homeostatic forces for deep sleep. Ana Ribeiro et al. (2007) in my lab set up experiments in which mice were fed only during the middle of the time they ordinarily would sleep, 8 hours before their usual period of maximal food intake. She showed that, yes, compared to controls who fed at the normal time, food-shifted mice became aroused before the altered feeding time and displayed more than five times the amount of movement during that (ordinarily sleeping) time. Further, this hunger-induced arousal was accompanied by activation specifically of neurons in a hypothalamic cell group which regulates food intake.

If indeed, the sudden and sensitive brain change from very low GA to high GA has the physical character of a phase transition. As proposed (Pfaff and Banavar, 2007), what nerve cell groups help to account for the suddenness of some of the transitions? Earlier chapters mentioned Clifford Saper's emphasis on pairs of structures showing mutual inhibitory relations with each other (reviewed, Saper et al., 2010). With optogenetics, Chung et al. (2017) generated the most recent evidence that the ventrolateral preoptic sleep-active neurons contribute to such yin/yang, flip-flop relations. In Saper's writing he emphasized hypothalamic cell groups and groups in the pons and midbrain. Equally important, thalamocortical and corticothalamic signaling have been emphasized by other neurophysiologists (e.g., Steriade, 2003).

Sleep Disruption. Of course, behavioral rhythms well-tuned to circadian rhythms are necessary for health. Without the deepest sleep – featuring the slowest EEG waves in the 0.5–4 per second range – coupled with REM sleep, psychological difficulties will ensue. Ilia Koratsoreos and Bruce McEwen found that certain deviations from the standard 12:12 light:dark cycle standard for laboratory mice caused physiological problems reminiscent of the metabolic syndrome: a set of conditions including abdominal obesity, high blood pressure, and high blood sugar, conditions that lead to diabetes and heart disease. Beyond the lab, the so-called "nickel and dime" Navy schedule (5 hours work,

10 hours off) was held partially responsible for Naval underperformance leading to accidents that damaged U.S. naval vessels. Eve Van Cauter's lab provides a clinical counterpart to Koratsoreos' and McEwen's results (Knutson and Van Cauter, pp. 287–304 in Pfaff and Kieffer, 2008): loss of normal sleep, as reported in clinical epidemiological studies, is associated with an increased risk of diabetes, failure to regulate appetite, and higher body-mass index (BMI). Van Cauter, a clinician with expertise in neuroendocrinology, argues that these sleep-related metabolic abnormalities derive from inaccuracies in the signaling of two neuropeptides: leptin (signaling from fat) and ghrelin (signaling from gastrointestinal lining). The U.S. navel problems, cited above, potentially find their explanation in the report "Sleep Deprivation and Vigilant Attention" by veteran sleep researcher David Dinges, at the University of Pennsylvania (Lim and Dinges, pp. 305–22, in Pfaff and Kieffer, 2008). Using his "psychomotor vigilance test," Dinges writes that sleep deprivation (i) slows responses, (ii) causes lapses of attention and errors of commission, (iii) magnifies the effect of on-task fatigue, and, as expected, (iv) demonstrates the effects of Alexander Borbely's second of two factors, the homeostatic drive on sleep.

Genetics. Knowledge of the genetics which contribute to sleep regulation (and sleep disorders) is growing rapidly. Emmanuel Mignot, a physician/scientist at Stanford Medical School cited above for his work on hypocretin, reviewed evidence for the genetic regulation of sleep which covered molecules previously suspected such as adenosine (which promotes sleep; caffeine blocks adenosine receptors), hypocretin, and other arousal-related neurotransmitters discussed in this book (Sehgal and Mignot, 2011). Sehgal and Mignot also cover intracellular signaling molecules which act downstream of these neurotransmitters and neuropeptides, including a protein kinase A pathway, an extracellular-regulated kinase (ERK) pathway, and others. Work with fruit flies revealed the gene *sleepless* which encodes a small protein that regulates a specific potassium channel. Obviously, circadian clock genes are involved. As reviewed in Sehgal and Mignot, several sleep-regulating genetic pathways are conserved between fruit flies and mammals. New work has been focused on genetic loci associated with disorders like sleep apnea and restless leg syndrome.

Forward genetics, the approach which leads from phenotype toward the genetic basis of that phenotype, applied to sleep required "recording patterns of sleep for two consecutive days in more than 8000 mice carrying genetic mutations that were randomly induced in one of their parents" identified two interesting mutations (summarized by Dijk and Winsky-Sommerer, 2016). Funato et al. (2016), who did the forward genetic work at the University of Tsukuba, Japan's "science city," found an RNA splicing mutation in a protein kinase gene which "caused a profound decrease in total wake time." A second line of mice which carried a "missense gain of function mutation" in a sodium leak channel reduced the amount of REM sleep; thus, the *sleepy* and *dreamless* mutations. The job now for neurobiologists is to figure out exactly why these mutations lead to the sleep phenotypes described.

Sleep Drive. Previous chapters covered neural circuitries contributing to sleep drive, e.g., chapters about the pons and the hypothalamus. Most prominent in these circuits are ventrolateral preoptic area neurons that are active during sleep (Sherin et al., 1996) produce the neuropeptide galanin (Gaus et al., 2002) and express the gene for the somnogen prostaglandin D (Mong et al., 2003a, b). Clifford Saper (2001) followed the lead of the classical sleep expert von Economo and the expert neuroanatomist Walle J. H. Nauta by visualizing relationships between these ventrolateral reoptic area neurons and wake-promoting nerve cell groups. Most importantly, he saw that mutually inhibitory relations between these two types of nerve cell groups, with certain time delays, would lead to the capacity for "relatively rapid and complete state transitions," sleep switches (Saper et al. 2010).

Traumatic Brain Injury

First there is the matter of definitions, as taken from the descriptions by Schiff and Plum (2000). Coma, a totally unconscious and unarousable brain state, includes unresponsiveness to internal or external stimuli. "Eyes are closed and even the most vigorous exogenous stimulation cannot evoke awakening." In contrast, in the vegetative state, we note the appearance of "irregular cyclic arousal (absent in the comatose patient) recovers without evidence of awareness of self or the environment."

The very first problem facing the neurologist examining a patient who suffered traumatic brain injury is to make an accurate diagnosis (Posner et al., 2007). Standardized scales for doing so were mentioned in Chapter 1, the most widely used being the revised Glasgow Coma Recovery Scale (CRS). Additionally, Stephen Laureys, professor of neurology at the University of Liege (Bodart et al., 2017), successfully used ^{18}F-fluorodeoxyglucose (FDG)-positron emission tomography (PET) to add precision by measuring brain regional metabolic activity. For example, the Laureys team used these metabolic measurements to complement the most sensitive behavioral approach (Wannez et al., 2017), the Coma Recovery Scale-Revised (CRS-R), to analyze results from minimally conscious state (MCS) patients. Some positive behavioral signs of low-level awareness are frequent: eye fixation, "visual pursuit, and reproducible movement to command." Other behaviors were rarely observed: "object localisation (reaching), object manipulation, intelligible verbalisation, and object recognition." Again, for diagnostic precision, the Laureys unit in Liege (Demertzi et al., 2015) used the CRS-R and positron emission tomography scanning for which functional connectivity was investigated for several networks in the default mode, frontoparietal, salience, auditory, sensorimotor, and visual. Statistical analyses of the results led to "a high discriminative capacity (>80%) for separating patients in a minimally conscious state and vegetative state/unresponsive wakefulness syndrome."

Jan Claassen, professor of neurology at Columbia's College of Physicians and Surgeons, has written widely about the use of state-of-the-art electroencephalography (EEG) for diagnostic purposes, with special attention to coma. In addition to the traditional frequency power spectrum, he measures coherence of wave activity across brain regions, EEG complexity, and phase/amplitude coupling as analytic tools. For example, Claassen et al. (2016) studied initially comatose patients following subarachnoid hemorrhage, some of whom had improved behaviorally. All patients were rated as aware, arousable, or still comatose. Then, with EEG, "central gamma, posterior alpha, and diffuse theta-delta oscillations differentiated patients who were arousable from those in coma. The simplest way of describing their results is to say that in coma, high frequency gamma waves are lost and low frequency delta waves are enhanced. Command following was characterized by a further increase in central gamma and posterior alpha." They concluded that distinctive EEG patterns added usefully to behavioral measurements in tracking the progress of these patients. Claassen et al. (2013) performed a systematic review of 42 studies, including comatose patients, and came away with the recommendation that EEG be used to detect ischemia in comatose patients and a variety of other conditions.

Further, the Laureys lab (2017) showed that high-density EEG, analyzed by graph theory, produced sets of metrics that should reduce misdiagnosis in patients with several types of disorders of consciousness. Following classification analysis, they can predict the "brain metabolism and 1-year clinical outcome of individual patients" and thus guide plans for further treatment.

Beyond the EEG, Rohaut and Naccache (2017) have recorded evoked potentials in the electrical activity of the cortex for further insight into the patient's level of consciousness. These were brain signals recorded in response to specific types of stimulation. The bottom line is that the conscious brain showed two specific peaks in the evoked potential in response to auditory stimuli that could be distinguished from responses during unconscious processing.

Additional precautions regarding diagnosis come from computing autonomic cardiac markers, such as heart rate (HR) and HR variability (HRV), and cardiac cycle phase shifts triggered by the processing of the auditory stimuli (Raimondo et al., 2017). The authors were able to distinguish MCS patients from other conditions by a phase shift of the cardiac cycle and other cardiac markers. They felt that their results "open a new window to evaluate patients with disorders of consciousness."

Edlow et al. (2017) wanted to better predict emergence of consciousness in patients with severe brain injury by adding task-based functional magnetic resonance imaging to EEG techniques. Amongst a variety of initial levels of behavioral performance of the 34 patients enrolled, complete absence of responses to language, music, and motor imagery was only observed in coma patients. Important was the novel report in this paper of "covert command following": (seen in the fMRI but not at bedside). Overall, the results showed that the combination of functional magnetic resonance imaging (fMRI) and EEG can detect command-following and higher-order cortical function in patients recovering from severe injury.

In the room at the Rockefeller University Hospital where Professor Nicholas Schiff examines high-end vegetative state patients whom he hopes will re-enter consciousness (in the Consortium for the Advanced Study of Brain Injury), I have witnessed traumatic brain injury patients who have been knocked to the pavement in a fight and cut down by a motor scooter, among other violent encounters. But not all vegetative state patients that Schiff targets for ameliorative treatments had experienced this kind of violent accident. In *Rights Come to Mind* (2015), Cornell professor of Medicine Joseph J. Fins cites unresponsiveness associated with a tracheotomy and lung infection, a blockage of a major artery in the brainstem and other cases. Fins regrets our relative "state of ignorance as we begin to classify brain injuries" (p. 27). Even with our new imaging equipment, "striking images of the brain remain descriptive and, as yet, do not provide a fully mechanistic account of disorders of consciousness."

As reviewed above, the most extreme state is coma: arousal and awareness are at zero. Coma is a temporary state; patients will die or will proceed to a vegetative state. In a high-end vegetative state (minimally conscious state), eyes will open, the patient can attend to stimuli, track stimuli, and follow commands beginning with the simplest commands with, hopefully, proceeding toward more complex commands. Cornell's professor Nicholas Schiff (2005) characterizes the high-end vegetative state condition known as the MCS by saying that an MCS patient can "demonstrate reliable but inconsistent evidence of self-awareness or the environment as demonstrated by verbal or gestural output" (p. 474). That is, the patient may sporadically speak or respond with a grin to something humorous, for example. In fact, from experiments with lab animals, I believe that emotional functions may be unusually resilient; in mice, fear learning was not damaged by anoxia, when other components of GA, motor activity, and sensory responsiveness were affected (Arrieta-Cruz et al., 2007).

There have been surprises. Adrian Owen and colleagues (2006) used fMRI to study a vegetative-state patient who, when imagining a particular activity, demonstrated activation in the part of the cerebral cortex responsible for such an activity. Later they raised broad questions about the full extent of cognitive and emotional capacities which remain in the brains of some vegetative state patients (Owen and Coleman, 2008a, b). Likewise, Schiff et al. (2005) were able to use "personalized narratives to elicit cortical activity in the superior and middle temporal gyrus." When the recordings were played backwards, the cortex of MCS patients "demonstrated markedly reduced responses."

Paths toward Consciousness. As mentioned, if a vegetative-state patient can show sporadic signs of awareness, language use, or command following, that patient may be designated as having arrived at a separate state: "minimally conscious." Schiff et al. (2007) treated a traumatic brain-injured patient, who had not been conscious for more than 6 years, in a double-blind alternating crossover study to determine the therapeutic effectiveness of electrical stimulation of the central thalamus. Very quickly upon the beginning of the stimulation, Schiff and his colleagues noted improvements in the patient's awareness: "abrupt changes in his CRS scores, longer periods of eye opening, and increased responsiveness to commands." Then, "functional object use and intelligible verbalization." The deep-brain stimulation followed On and Off phases. What I found most encouraging was the gradual improvement in arousal and awareness during the "off" phases, suggesting that, with time, the effect of the stimulation could, increasingly, carry over to non-stimulation time periods.

It is interesting that another recent report (Adams et al., 2016) focused on the sleep dynamics of a TBI patient who had been in a minimally conscious state for 21 years. In terms of neurophysiology, the authors pointed out that "two key elements of healthy sleep, spindles and slow waves, are generated via thalamocortical feedback loops that prominently involve the neurons within the central thalamus." Central thalamic stimulation did not improve this patient's overall behavioral profile. Before central thalamic stimulation the patient showed abnormal mixing of EEG-measured sleep features. Normalization of sleep architecture following central thalamic stimulation included both an improved segregation of sleep features according to stages and the emergence of REM sleep.

Schiff (2010) conceived of a "mesocircuit" model to account for recoveries of consciousness after brain injury – that is, not a cell-and-neighboring-cell "microcircuit," and not a whole brain "macrocircuit." His model had two purposes. First, he had to account for the success of central thalamic stimulation. Second, he had to explain the surprising response of some MCS patients to the sleeping medication, zolpidem. His model features widespread excitatory projections from central thalamus to cortex and, importantly, feedback through the basal ganglia to the thalamus. Two successive inhibitory synapses in the model, on the way back through the basal ganglia to thalamus, can explain the zolpidem effect by invoking disinhibition.

In postcardiac-arrest patients, Forgacs et al. (2017) concentrated on EEG spectral features corresponding to higher levels of anterior forebrain corticothalamic integrity correlated with higher levels of consciousness and favorable clinical outcome. The most interesting point of the Forgacs study lay in the fact that these were *acute* post-cardiac arrest patients and that levels of EEG normality corresponding to anterior forebrain integrity predicted the eventual outcome at the time of hospital discharge. Schiff et al. (2013) examined microelectrode recording results in non-human primate thalamus to understand short-term adjustments of attentional effort. Their findings indicated that "central thalamic neurons regulate task performance through brief changes in firing rates and spectral power changes during task-relevant short-term shifts of attentional effort." With regard to the data I have reviewed with respect to low-road and high-road contributions to consciousness, it appears that thalamocortical and corticothalamic connections are crucial in humans and non-human primates for arousal and attention to task-relevant stimuli, while basal forebrain neurons make their major contributions in lower animals with respect to changes in behavioral state.

Other forms of brain stimulation may also be helpful. The Laureys lab used repeated transcranial direct current stimulation (Thibaut et al., 2017) over the prefrontal cortex and observed a highly significant improvement in the CRS. Whether this is a specific effect that fits closely with the thalamocortical phenomena remains open to question. Finally, Schiff (2016) interprets success with central thalamic stimulation as energizing an "anterior forebrain mesocircuit" required for consciousness. Measures of cerebral metabolism (Fridman et al., 2014) using [(18)F]-fluorodeoxyglucose with brain-injured patients compared to controls support this point of view.

One of the interesting consequences of central thalamic stimulation could be theorized to involve increased coupling among cortical systems. Mathematician and neurologist Jonathan Victor explored this possibility computationally (Drover et al., 2010). Drover and Victor found answers that depended on exactly how thalamocortical relations are conceived: coupling via the thalamic reticular nucleus, compared to coupling via other relay nuclei. With the former, some computational solutions showed "distant cortical regions mainly in the same activity level," others just the opposite. With the latter, these striking contrasts were not obtained. Victor's work was followed up by Michael Halassa (Nakajima and Halassa, 2017), who reviewed current evidence that thalamocortical connections serve to regulate connectivity among cortical regions. As opposed to classical summaries of visual image processing and as opposed to GA, Halassa proposes an intermediate concept of "directed arousal states" which connect the power of GA to specific visual image processing.

As you would expect, the tragedies of traumatic brain injury have gained the attention of basic neuroscientists who work with laboratory animals. At the 2017 meeting of the Society for Neuroscience, several labs reported struggling to produce severe behavioral deficits following injuries to the mouse brain. Previously, in my lab, graduate student Amy Wells Quinkert (2010, 2012; Tabansky et al., 2014) had extended Schiff's clinical work to mice with the predicted results. More interesting is Baker et al.'s (2016) work with non-human primates. Central thalamic deep-brain stimulation, in a location-specific manner, enhanced GA and improved cognitive performance. The authors were able to shape the central thalamic electric field in three-dimensional space, allowing the animals to do better on visual/motor tasks, correlated with changes in electrical activity in the frontal cortex and basal ganglia

Finally, Joseph Fins (2015) puts everything in perspective (see Chapter 9) when he puts the MCS patients' experiences in the context of their families' trauma, and when he examines the ethics not only of treating MCS patients but, importantly, of *not* attending to the medical needs of MCS patients.

Summary

Modern electrophysiological and imaging techniques have led to tremendous progress in diagnosing and understanding severe brain injuries. First steps toward amelioration have been undertaken and are underway. Among the three low-GA states covered in this chapter, traumatic brain injury represents the tragic case.

Major Features of GA Mechanisms. In retrospect, it is easy to see how the reduction of some of the major features of GA mechanisms account for the loss of consciousness following traumatic brain injury, and anesthesia as well. First the long A/P, L systems I have emphasized would be interrupted at least in part, and at the same time overall connectivity would be reduced. With these losses the essence of "integration," identical signals being sent over long (potentially scale-free) neuronal systems would also disappear. Thus, loss of consciousness is over-determined.

Chapter 9

Roots of Consciousness and Its Disorders

Consciousness is too important to be left to philosophers. Consciousness, termed "the hard problem" by neurologists, is in colloquial English often be taken to mean "awake" and "self-aware."

Nevertheless, serious scholars who are not scientists seem to be writing about consciousness more frequently than ever before. So it seems necessary for me to briefly represent their views, to contrast subjectivity of philosophy of consciousness with the objectivity of the scientific method. Moreover, the odd scientist who has won a Nobel Prize will join the fray, as noted below.

Background. "Consciousness" is a favorite topic of philosophers, who often use physiological, and indeed neurological data to craft arguments about how we perceive ourselves and the world – that is, what it means to be self-aware or awake. Yet invariably, such arguments extrapolate from the science that they cite; hard data are often obscured in speculations that drift far from what science actually knows. Consciousness, in the philosophical sense, is only a concept or, rather, an array of concepts that are at least in part linguistically constructed. The concept(s) can be fascinating – and frequently are provocative – but they make no difference when doctors try to resuscitate someone after a drug-induced coma. They make no difference to the ordinary act of waking up every morning, which in fact, as we saw in Chapter 8, is a complex feat.

Of course, my concern is less expansive, more elementary, than what philosophy is able to encompass. But by the same token, this book may go further in addressing the question of how the human body actually transitions into consciousness. Consciousness, in a scientific sense, may never be exactly the same as philosophical consciousness. It is not necessarily even a singular predicate to it, since (as will emerge) philosophers have created many different notions of how we register any experience of ourselves and others. This book contrasts the hard science of how our brains emerge into consciousness, with its philosophical counterpart, so as to demonstrate why an understanding of that science will be determinative for medical practice. By extension, this chapter will also give a sense of what science still needs to learn about consciousness, and the directions that some cutting-edge works are taking.

Neuroscientists Weigh In

Discussions of consciousness that have received wide attention among neuroscientists have been published by the Nobel laureate Francis Crick and Christof Koch (2003, and Metzinger, 2002, p. 103), perhaps because of Crick's fame in discovering DNA and RNA, and Koch's recognition for his work on the visual cortex. Surprisingly, they seem to opine that "we are not directly aware of the outer world of sensory events, nor are we directly aware of our inner world of thoughts, intentions and planning" (p. 109). What we do know are the computations performed by our nervous system upon such inputs. This formulation reminds me of the many demonstrations by Richard Held, professor at MIT, that in order to respond to variations in our physical world we must perform active movements in that space. Koch and Crick had lots of ideas, comprehensive knowledge of the relevant literature, great expertise in the primate visual cortex, but, as far as I can tell, no coherent theory.

Another Nobel prizewinner, Gerald Edelman, and neuroscientist Giulio Tononi (1998, see also Sporns et al., 2000), and Metzinger (p. 139), wrote clearly about the assumptions involved when investigating consciousness. The "physics assumption" states that conventional physical processes are sufficient to explain consciousness. The "evolutionary assumption" says that consciousness evolved like other biological functions. I will discuss the evolutionary approach below. The "qualia assumption" admits subjectivity as an essential property of consciousness. But in terms of an explanation of consciousness, the authors' reference to a dynamic core looks a bit mystical to me. Nonetheless, they also emphasize "that for conscious experience to occur, the rapid integration of the activity of distributed brain regions through reentrant interactions is required" (p. 149). That emphasis is well in accord with the major themes of this book.

Neuroscientist Joseph LeDoux (LeDoux and Brown, 2017) has proposed a new approach to consciousness that is intended to account for all forms of fear awareness, from anticipation of physical pain to existential panic. Cortical networks are necessary for all forms of consciousness, but emotional experience subtends different kinds of inputs to those networks than nonemotional experience. These are nonconscious inputs from subcortical structures whose neurons manage reflex emotional responses. This is what LeDoux calls his "higher-order" theory because emotional information is re-represented; it seems well in accord with modern neuroscience.

Philosophers Must Deal with Subjectivity

This book focuses on those aspects of consciousness most approachable through neuroscientific techniques. In the previous chapters, I have been concerned with mechanisms that support the earliest steps of rising from deep anesthesia, deep sleep, or the effects of traumatic brain injury: paths toward consciousness. But one crucial aspect of consciousness is the state of being self-aware, commonly referred to as subjectivity.

The dictionary states that "subjectivity" means "arising from within, or belonging strictly to the individual." For Thomas Metzinger (2002), a professor of Philosophy at University of Osnabruck in Germany, consciousness is essentially a *subjective* target of inquiry. "Conscious experience, under standard conditions is always tied to an individual, first-person perspective" (p. 1). What he thinks he is looking for is a "strict and systematic correlation between a certain brain property" and "a subjectively experienced phenomenal property" (p. 4). He understands that there may be no causal relationship between the two, directly or indirectly.

The essential *subjectivity* inherent in the study of consciousness also comes to the fore when you consider Zen Buddhism: "Zen always aims at grasping the central fact of life, which can never be brought to the dissecting table of the intellect" (Suzuki, 1960, 51). This subjectivity, of course, is why I mention other scholars' treatments of various aspects of consciousness, but do not attempt analyses of my own, intellectual, or neuroscientific.

Several Prominent Philosophers' Attempts

In a historical chapter, Ansgar Beckermann (Metzinger, p. 41) harked back to arguments between biological mechanists, who held that the functions of living organisms could be explained mechanistically like clocks, and vitalists, who felt they needed to postulate "some special nonphysical substance in order to explain life." He contrasts two statements (p. 51): (1) pain in humans is identical to C-fiber firing; and (2) temperature in ideal gases is identical to the mean kinetic energy of their molecules. For reasons I do not understand, some philosophers say they are not the same, thus claiming that kinetic energy completely explains temperature, whereas he can *conceive* not feeling pain even though his C-fibers are firing. Pain has a qualitative character, the concept of which goes beyond C-fibers.

David Chalmers, professor of Philosophy at the University of Arizona, suggests that when the "neural correlate of consciousness" turns on, "your consciousness turns on in a corresponding way" (Metzinger, p. 17). The formal definition used at a Consciousness conference stated "a neural correlate of consciousness is a specific system in the brain whose activity correlates directly with states of conscious experience." Chalmers holds out the possibility that such correlated neuronal activity might be sufficient for conscious experience, but no proof of such sufficiency is available. The anterior/posterior, longitudinal (A/P, L) systems that I have discussed in this book are distributed widely enough in the brain that neither philosopher nor neurophysiologist could prove or disprove Chalmers' proposition of neural correlate sufficiency.

In Revonsuo's steps toward a biological research program on consciousness, he lists several problems to face, but the one (Metzinger, p. 60) that resonated with me is the measurement problem. He wants to "see" consciousness in some of our brain scanning techniques.

One of the premier philosophers of consciousness in recent decades is Daniel C. Dennett, professor at Tufts University. In *Consciousness Explained*, he states that "human consciousness is just about the last surviving mystery" (p. 21). He states that "we are still in a terrible muddle" (p. 22). After posing several tasks and entering several reflections intended to guide us, he startled me by imagining that artificial brains might "at least in principle" have all the functions of human brains, including, I infer, consciousness. But he celebrates consciousness without explaining it. He is against mind–brain dualism – the supposition that mind and brain must be considered as two separate entities – which, for reasons I don't understand, he calls "fundamentally antiscientific."

Dennett scrupulously lists steps that could go into the development of consciousness, from the simple ability to be warned by a dangerous stimulus, through "short-range anticipation" (p. 178) through other neurophysiological steps to mechanisms of cultural evolution. This biological approach can be contrasted with cultural evolution, which is said by geneticist Richard Dawkins, among others, to depend on the spread of "memes": a word that is supposed to play on the sounds of the words "genes" and "mimic." A meme is any cultural element that can be passed from one individual to another, e.g., by imitation.

And now we get to Dennett's big finale. For him, "Human consciousness is itself a huge complex of memes ... forming a virtual machine that vastly enhances the underlying powers of the organic hardware on which it runs" (p. 210). I simply do not understand how a statement like this moves neuroscience forward.

Philosopher Nick Humphrey (1992) also wants to explain "coming to," as from a deep sleep. He sees the "truth about consciousness – that it is indeed the product of a highly improbable bit of biological engineering" (p. 6). He takes for granted that consciousness must be "helping the organism to survive and reproduce" and therefore must reveal its presence at the level of behavior. However, the effects of conscious-like phenomena may be "more or less important for different kinds of animals," thus "pushing the evolution of consciousness along species specific lines" (p. 15). A conscious animal will have advantages over what Humphrey calls "psychological zombies," perhaps because they will have specific interests, care about things, and have goals they have set for themselves (p. 72). Consciousness "makes life more worth living" (p. 75).

In order to achieve a comprehensive theory, some philosophers throw the brain overboard and concentrate on the mental phenomena for their own sake. Christopher Hill and Ned Block are two tremendously learned philosophers. Hill, professor of philosophy at Brown University (Hill, 2009), considers that many scholars have distinguished no less than five types of consciousness: (i) agent consciousness, in which an agent is losing or regaining consciousness; (ii) propositional consciousness, which implies awareness of some factual knowledge; (iii) introspective consciousness, with which we reflect on our own and others' states of awareness; (iv) relational consciousness, which uses the "conscious of" construction; and (v) phenomenal consciousness, which includes perceptual appreciation of "qualitative characteristics as pain and the taste of oranges." To these, Hill adds (vi) experiential consciousness, which sounds intuitively attractive but vague. Hill expands his initial definition of experiential consciousness by saying (p. 10) "When you consider an experiential state introspectively, are you aware of the intrinsic phosphorescence that the state shares with all other experiences?" He concludes (p. 12) "that experiences are mental events that participate in certain distinctive ways in the stream of higher level cognitive activity." I must admit Hill's excursions into the philosophy of mind deal with sophisticated features of conscious thought far more mentally oriented than anything in this book. By analogy to auto mechanics, Hill explains the carburetors and the transmissions of racing Ferraris, while I am just trying to get the motor started – any motor.

Ned Block is a professor of philosophy at New York University. I want philosophers to make things clear, but over the years I have encountered his writing and come away confused. Wanting to figure out what Block's (2007) "functionalism" means, I read (p. 17) "According to functionalism, the nature of a mental state is just like the nature of an automaton state – that is, constituted by its relations to other states and to inputs and outputs. All there is to S1 is that being in it and getting a '1' input results in such and such, etc. According to functionalism, all there is to being in pain is that it disposes you to say 'ouch.'" And there are subdivisions of functionalism (p. 27): computation-representation functionalism ("providing a computer program for the mind"); functional analysis (a research strategy and a consequent type of explanation that "explains the working of the system in terms of the capacities of the parts and the way the parts are integrated with one another"); and metaphysical functionalism (mental states are functional states). Does this help? Beyond my difficulty with that writing, I am drowning in "isms." As a partial list: functionalism, representationism, social constructivism, behaviorism, physicalism. Renaming philosophical approaches to problems as "isms" does not clarify.

Mind–Body Problem

What of the "mind–body problem," which is in effect the "mind–brain" problem? Considered by the seventeenth-century French philosopher Rene Descartes, among others, this scholarly exercise wrestles with causal relations between mind and body taken separately. The mind–body–brain problem asks you to determine whether the mind is co-extensive with the brain or something separate. Are experiential phenomena separate from physical phenomena?

This book does not pay much attention to the mind–brain problem because it likely leads to a useless paradox. When any mind (such as yours or mine) considers the mind–body problem or the mind–brain problem, we run into troublesome difficulties of self-reference. I take my lesson from the twentieth-century British logician and mathematician Bertrand Russell. Consider his paradoxes of self-reference: "This sentence is a lie." Or the formulation used by the Cretan philosopher Epimenides, and later by Saint Jerome: "All men are liars." Or another paradox proposed by Russell: "The barber is the one who shaves all those, and those only, who do not shave themselves." The question is, does the barber shave himself? There is no non-paradoxical answer to this question. Likewise, "True or false: This sentence is false." And also, "If a man tries to fail and succeeds, which did he do?" Summing up, I fear that the "mind–brain" problem leads to a paradox of self-reference and therefore is not useful to pursue.

I reach this conclusion with caution because there are times when a paradox is exactly what a field of science needs. A productive paradox can stimulate scientists to examine, in a creative fashion, the underpinnings of their field. Noson Yonofsky (2016) gives examples. Light can act both as a wave and a particle. "This duality ushers a whole new dimension into science" (p. 166). Indeed, as Yonofsky says, "There are reasons to believe that there is a lot more 'out there' that we cannot know than what we can know" (p. 172). But I and many others have been thinking about the mind–brain problem for more than 50 years, and it has not yet yielded insight.

Evolution

Gebhard Roth, of the Brain Research Institute in the University of Bremen, Germany, thinks of our species in an evolutionarily "nested" sense, that is, taxonomically placed among chimpanzees, apes, primates, and, most broadly, mammals (Metzinger, p. 77). In his view, it is not possible to parse nearness or absence of consciousness among various biological forms because we are not even sure about our closest relatives.

As a basis for comparison among species, he suggests perhaps zeroing in on specific brain region. For Roth, everything points to the cerebral cortex as necessary for full consciousness. Having said that, what are the contributions of various cortical regions? Much writing has been devoted to the relative importance of cortical regions with special emphasis on the associative cortex because it might contribute more to certain forms of consciousness than primary sensory or motor cortex.

A different approach would ask: what are some cognitive functions that, for humans, would require consciousness, and which animals have (some of) those functions? Credibly, he highlights "comprehension of underlying mechanisms" – for example, great apes using tools. Also, he suggests "theory of mind," the ability to understand another's knowledge and intentions. Great apes and chimps show this ability. "Anticipation of future events" is shown by great apes. Roth (p. 84) also includes "self-recognition in a mirror," of which great apes and dolphins are capable. "Understanding and using simple syntactical language" also counts according to Roth, another capability of great apes and dolphins.

Comparisons among species are shaky in some respects because they depend on how intensively experiments have tried to bring out various cognitive abilities. A rule of thumb among ethologists would state that an animal can do everything you know it can, and then some.

Nick Humphrey's approach to the evolution of consciousness is different. For Humphrey, a theoretical psychologist at the New School and London School of Economics, it "is all in the senses" – "nothing is in the mind that was not first in the senses." Humphrey (1992) wants to know what it is to have sensations. He gives five indicia (p. 132): (i) sensations belong to the subject, the individual person; (ii) they are tied to a location, a body space; (iii) they are sensory modality specific (e.g., vision as opposed to audition); (iv) they are "present tense"; and (v) they are "self-characterizing" – "each sensation tells its own story" and we know what its properties are.

Unfortunately, Humphrey waxes metaphoric. He talks about turning "the water of the physical brain into the wine of consciousness." He speaks of reverberating cerebral sentiments (p. 221). This does not represent a comprehensive theory.

I come away from Humphrey's work with the strategic guess that the evolution of consciousness has proceeded apace with the evolution of the neocortex. No surprises there. But this book shows the intricacy of the lower brainstem systems whose scaling properties offer the volume of signaling that enables the neocortex to do its job.

Neurological Approaches and Considerations

As noted, early in the twentieth century, Frederic Bremer, a Belgian neurologist, made transections of the brainstems of cats and observed the animals' capacities for sleeping and waking. Transecting at the bottom of the brainstem did not have an effect on arousal, but transecting so as to separate the forebrain from the brainstem caused what appeared to be deep sleep-like state. Thus began a long tradition of studies on state changes in the CNS. According to Giacino et al. (2014) "The concept of consciousness continues to defy definition." The definition of a comatose state, as described by neurologist Adam Zeman (2002), comprises an absolute loss of consciousness due "to extensive damage to the hemispheres or to the thalamus" (p. 133). Such a state might be caused by a terrible head injury, a loss of blood supply, or, simply, a loss of oxygen. Such brain damage that affects states of consciousness is as appalling as any disease because it destroys mental life and one's sense of self. As presented by Cornell professor of neurology, Nicholas Schiff (Schiff and Plum, 2000) comatose states are, by definition, not permanent. Patients either die or they progress to a vegetative state, in which they do not show sustained purposeful movements or language comprehension, but do have sleep–wake cycles, visceral and autonomic functions, and spinal reflexes (Laureys, 2016a, b). In earlier years, some thought of a persistent vegetative state as permanent. Now, however, a subset of vegetative-state patients is recognized as displaying sporadic signs of self-awareness or of its environment (Schiff et al., 2005). These patients have been diagnosed as living in a "minimally conscious state" and show cortical electroencephalographic (EEG) responses to auditory linguistic stimulation. Such patients are prime candidates for therapeutic interventions.

Global Neuronal Workspace. Stanislas Dehaene et al. (2001a, b) and Dehaene and Christen (2011) have contributed a model of consciousness that he calls the Global Neuronal Workspace (GNW). The main idea is that specific cognitive functions such as attentional systems, perceptual systems, long-term memories, and evaluative systems all feed into the GNW which is a higher order, unified space of neuroanatomically distributed neurons characterized by extremely high connectivity in the cortex. This picture is sympathetic to the scale-free systems I mentioned in Chapter 2. Heightened arousal, necessary for high vigilance, would decrease "the threshold for global ignition of the GNW." One might ask, logically, about the causal relations between the GNW and consciousness. Is an active GNW necessary for consciousness, the reverse, or both?

EEG Gamma Wave Synchrony. Neuroscientists are on the hunt for the features of cerebral cortex electrical activity that are necessary for consciousness. In terms of activity, a certain class of high-frequency wave activity is of special interest. EEG waves in the frequency range of 35–58 waves per second (Hz), gamma waves, are often associated with active cognitive processing. Cantero and Atienza (2005) have presented evidence of "state-dependent synchrony" in recording gamma oscillations as a feature of the waking, active brain. Likewise, Doesburg et al. (2008), knowing that "Gamma-band synchronization has been proposed to be a mechanism for the functional integration of neural populations," observed such synchronization in the visual cortex during a task of visual attention. Buzsáki and Schomburg (2015) have presented the advantages and cautions of considering gamma rhythm synchrony as evidence of coupling among different regions of the forebrain, and Ray and Maunsell (2015) have considered the technical problems of interpretation of gamma rhythm coupling. As an educated reader of that literature, I feel that the authors studying about gamma-band synchronization really have something, but that both the methodology and the conceptualization need to be refined if the subject is going to contribute to our understanding of consciousness.

Default Mode Network(s). Another interesting aspect of human cortex electrical activity is in Raichle et al. (2001), describing the so-called "Default Mode Network" which is defined as a unique group of cortical regions that are active when there is no special task for the subject to do, but in which activity is decreased during performance of a wide range of cognitive tasks. Snyder (2016) has reviewed this area of work comprehensively and has concluded that activity in such a network depends on the level of CNS arousal being decreased in slow-wave sleep and anesthesia. There is a significant likelihood, in my view, that the Default Mode Network has something to do with our underlying sense of awareness when we are not doing a specific task. A useful analogy might be to an automobile engine idling when the car's transmission is not in gear and the car is not going anyplace. And then, for tasks involving specific sensory systems, Snyder (2016) reviews the evidence for "Resting State" systems devoted to particular sensory modalities.

Cerebral Cortical Hubs. Further, we must ask about the nature of the cerebral cortex connectivity that is optimal for the human's conscious performance. Not all connections are equal. Buckner et al. (2009) consider that "some brain areas act as *hubs* (italics mine) interconnecting distinct, functionally specialized systems." Buckner's functional magnetic resonance imaging (fMRI) datasets demonstrated hubs throughout association cortex – i.e., cortex outside primary sensory and motor controlling regions. Many of these hubs were previously implicated as components of the default network just cited. Buckner thinks that these hubs comprise "a stable property of cortical network architecture." Likewise, Hagmann et al. (2008) used a non-invasive imaging method to map pathways within and across cortical hemispheres in individual human participants. Their results revealed "brain regions within a structural core share high degree and strength" of connectedness, and so they likely comprise hubs of cerebral cortical activity.

Recently, Hudson et al. (2014) used electrophysiological recordings to analyze recovery from pharmacologically induced coma – deep anesthesia, consciousness at zero – to show that the recovery of neuronal activity does not follow a smooth monotonic curve that simply reflects decreasing concentration of anesthetic. Instead, recovering neuronal activity forms discrete metastable states, "dynamic hubs," persistent on the scale of minutes. To ultimately enter the activity state compatible with consciousness, the brain must first *pass through these hubs* in an orderly fashion. Whether these hubs defined by the dynamics of electrical activity are related to the connectivity hubs referred to above remains an open question, although the correspondence of one to the other presents an attractive thought.

Ethical Questions about Disorders of Consciousness

Joseph Fins, professor of medicine, health care policy, medicine in psychiatry and medical ethics at Weill Cornell Medical College, has laid out major issues in the identification and treatment of patients with disorders of consciousness in his book *Rights Come to Mind* (2015). First, he gives a range of examples, not at all limited to professional football's traumatic brain injuries that can lead to serious problems: in one case a young woman with a blockage in a major artery in her brainstem. Then he charts the diagnosis of states above the level of coma which the neurologist encounters. In particular, from the notion of a "vegetative state" – "wakefulness without awareness" (p. 35) – or, worse, persistent or permanent vegetative state, there had to evolve a new idea that would lead to recognition of "a group of individuals who had appeared unconscious but were not in a vegetative state, meaning that they retained some conscious awareness. Their awareness fluctuated ..." (p. 72). These were patients who sporadically would show some awareness of their environment, or even briefly interact with their doctor. Thus emerged the concept of the "minimally conscious state" and this recognition led to the breakthrough for a single-patient clinical trial led by Nicholas Schiff, professor of neurology at Cornell (see Chapter 6). As a neuroscientist, I note that the essence of this clinical recognition lay in the doctors' keen attention to the patients' behavior rather than in the interpretation of fMRI, the benefits of which are routinely overstated due to its lack of adequate spatial resolution, temporal resolution, and inability to distinguish excitatory neurons from inhibitory neurons. Doctors such as Schiff and Fin also pay keen attention to the "centrality of ethics" (p. 217) to the science of consciousness.

Professor Fins has issued a *cri de coeur* for attention to and advocacy concerning patients with disorders of consciousness. Patients' families cannot do it by themselves. They become fatigued and depressed. In Fins' view, building on the Americans with Disabilities Act, activists can "affirm consciousness as a right that must be recognized, respected and enabled" (p. 309).

Outlook

Massive resources are being brought to bear on questions concerning how the human cerebral cortex participates in mental activities that we call "consciousness." Former President Barack Obama's BRAIN (Brain Research through Advancing Innovative Neurotechnologies) Initiative is developing new analytic tools. Already, new scanning techniques, neuroanatomical approaches, and electrical recording programs are contributing to the completion of what are termed the connectome of the human brain. The Chan-Zuckerberg initiative that lubricates interactions among three universities – Stanford, University of California at Berkeley, and UCSF – will yield collaborative results which will be used widely. There is no telling what these massive initiatives will come up with, in regards to consciousness.

Chapter 10

A Vertically Integrated System

The visible represents an expression of the invisible. (Museum of Art, Hubei Province, China).

Observable, quantifiable behaviors are products of neuronal phenomena (at the molecular and physiological levels) which neuroscientists seek to understand and, ultimately, demonstrate – sometimes in necessarily novel ways. One of these is by employing reverse engineering, that is, by analyzing arousal mechanisms with the intention of deducing design features. In this vein, I sought to reverse engineer brain arousal mechanisms by reframing a vital question about the activation of behavior. This book employed a formulation not previously used: *"Why does any animal or human do anything at all?"* What are the mechanisms for initiating explicit, observable behaviors?

To answer the italicized question, this book surveys hundreds of papers which illuminate this topic, including some from my lab. Several key points emerged from this study.

First, I have proposed that the major features of brain arousal mechanisms comprise an Anterior/Posterior Longitudinal (A/P, L) ladder-like network. Since arousal network structure is likely to predict aspects of arousal network function, the second key point noted below is that this network may have "scale-free" properties. That means that a frequency distribution of the number of connections per neuron, in a log–log plot, would be a straight line.

Second, reticular formation neurons often project locally, as well as over medium and very large distances. As a result, the signal-receiving neurons over substantial lengths in the A/P axis of the GA system have greater capacities for coordination among their activities. This is the essence of neural integration. This idea of identical signals transmitted over very short, medium, and very long distances is sketched in Figure 6.1. If a scale-free network structure does to some extent imply function, then it fits perfectly with the behavioral data sketched in Figure 1.1.

Third, the overall amount of connectivity in arousal networks (scale-free or not) is higher than previously expected – connections proliferate among myencephalon (medulla), metencephalon (pons), mesencephalon (midbrain), diencephalon (both hypothalamus and thalamus), and telencephalon. High degrees of connectivity serve requirements for *combinations* of inputs from other modules. One obvious example would come in the central thalamus, receiving inputs from both the pedunculopontine nucleus in the pons and NGC neurons in the medulla. Not only that, but certain unique NGC neurons in the medullary reticular formation, those which express endothelial nitric oxide synthase (eNOS), appear to be part of a "vertically integrated" system in which, by virtue of their transcriptome and their proximity to blood vessels, these eNOS neurons may be able to control their own blood supply (Tabansky et al., 2018). As an analogy, Ford Motor Company may be "vertically integrated" if it owns its own automobile parts suppliers, and thus can respond adaptively and quickly to production challenges. In turn, my lab presented molecular evidence that these unique NGC neurons could affect their own extracellular matrix and, because of their proximity to capillaries, could increase their caliber by releasing nitric oxide in response to novelty in the environment (Tabansky et al., 2018).

Fourth, as mentioned, the idea of "integration" means the formation of a more complete, coordinated entity from disparate parts. The A/P, L system suggested here is integrated because, in part, of very large cells with very long axons sending identical messages to different levels of the neuraxis. That is, thinking of the medullary NGC neurons as the "master cells" of GA, one can see that their long-distance signaling in a scale-free network provides the very essence of integration, the rendering of one coherent arousal system from many disparate parts.

These NGC neurons are "first responders." Their job is to react in an adaptive fashion to all levels of environmental inputs, from alerting to alarming situations. Their dendrites spread wide. They respond to every sensory modality tested. Their descending axons influence motor neurons bilaterally at all levels of the spinal cord. Their ascending axons impact the nearby pons, but also the midbrain, central thalamus, hypothalamus, and distant basal forebrain. They can fire at high frequencies. Putting all of these facts together indicates the high channel capacity of NGC neurons, their ability to take in large amounts of information, and to send highly informative signals to a large number of neuronal groups. One suspects that the wide range of axonal links between NGC neurons could contribute to the scale-free behavior over three orders of magnitude, typical of a phase transition, observed by Alex Proekt in my lab's GA assay (Proekt et al., 2012). As noted (Tabansky et al., 2018), four converging lines of evidence point to the ability of some NGC neurons to regulate their own blood supply, another example of vertical integration. It is logical to think about these four points in the context of the current excitement about network theory.

Network Theory. Chapters 1 and 2 introduced research that lends itself to "reverse engineering" the A/P, L GA system (Figure 6.1). Network theory may add insight about how GA works. Considering the largest reticular formation neurons – certainly including NGC (Chapter 2) – with tremendously large numbers of connections, as well as the excess of small neurons with only local connections, we might be dealing with a scale-free GA system (Barabasi, 2009; for electrophysiological data, see He, 2014). Kaiser (2011) examined the question of whether human neuronal circuits are really scale-free and said "yes" for circuits in the cortex and hippocampus, albeit with different exponents in the equation below.

A scale-free net can be described by a simple exponential equation:

$$P(C) \sim \text{approximately } kC^{-\alpha} \tag{10.1}$$

That is, the probability of a neuron's having a certain number of connections approximately proportional to that number of connections (C) raised to the (−)alpha power.

Albert-Lazlo and Barabasi (Barabasi and Albert, 1999) believe that these interesting scale-free networks grow as such, due to the tendency of new hubs (or nodes), which are very well connected preferentially to draw in new connections as the network grows (reviewed, Bullmore and Sporns, 2009). Further, Barabasi (Li et al., 2017) has recently argued that networks whose structures can change over time, as brain networks can, are controllable, and are more efficient than static networks.

Surely this type of system, in the brain, uses the largest reticular formation neurons, notably NGC, to send identical messages to a wide range of neuronal targets stretching from the lowest spinal cord to the thalamus and basal forebrain. *Again, that is what integration means, i.e. taking many disparate signals and states and molding them to a singular initiative.*

In such a network, NGC neurons certainly comprise what network theorists call a "hub" or "node" (Figure 6.1). Control system engineer, Cal Tech professor John Doyle, calls the fan-in/ fan-out system typified by NGC neurons a "bowtie" network, a design which he considers ideal (Csete and Doyle, 2004).

What potentially are the other functional implications of the GA system comprising a scale-free network, if indeed the network is scale-free? One possibility is that the system achieves what network theorists call criticality, which includes the ability to make rapid and adaptive responses to tiny changes in inputs. Pfaff and Banavar (2007) theorized that such phase transitions characterize CNS arousal systems. Data from the Human Connectome Project subsequently have yielded evidence of scale-invariance (Taylor et al., 2017). Likewise, Marcelo Magnasco et al. (2009) have written about an elegant neuronal net to achieve criticality: When recording human cortical electrical activity, Alonso et al. (2014) stated that "while the subject is awake, many modes of neuronal activity oscillations are found at the edge of instability." Hesse and Gross (2014) agree with Magnasco that "As expected at criticality, neuronal avalanches show further scale-free properties," but they do not convincingly link this dynamic functionality to the formation of a scale-free network.

Gyorgy Buzsaki (2006) has considered both sides of the issue concerning whether scale-free networks offer unexpected control system advantages or, instead, risk creating crippling susceptibilities. On the one hand, he feels that an explicit implication of a scale-free network is that the network's dynamics will achieve "self-organized criticality" (p. 128) which would generate response capacities that are quick and flexible. On the other hand, since the major hubs with many connections, such as NGC, "dictate the action" (p. 41), damage to them would cripple the system, and their infection by abnormal activity rhythms could lead to an epidemic in the entire system (Stam, 2014; Mitra et al., 2017). Regarding NGC, neurosurgeons do not go there for this type of reason. They do not take the risk of surgery in this brain region.

Chapter 6 introduced the notion of a scale-free network. As mentioned, this means that a small number of neurons have very large numbers of connections, and large numbers of neurons have very small numbers of connections. In a frequency distribution plot on log–log axes, with numbers of connections on the X-axis and the number of neurons with such connections on the Y-axis, the plot comes to approximately a straight line. As summarized by Olaf Sporns (2011), such networks have a low degree of randomness, the highest degree of heterogeneity, and low "modularity" (meaning segmentation by function). These properties fit what we neuroscientists need for GA pathways. These network properties have been invoked in functional "criticality" as theorized by Pfaff and Banavar (2007) and by Marcelo Magnasco (above) in the tradition of the physicist Chris Langton (1990). Langton surmised that the information processing ability of a network would be maximized when the network is poised near the transition from chaos to orderly dynamics, "in a critical state." Sporns agrees that "the critical dynamic regime has many properties that are highly desirable for neural information-processing systems" and are "associated with maximal information transfer" (p. 270). The "long range correlations" he cites as typical of the critical network state are precisely what is achieved in the brainstem by the A/P, L reticular neurons that are highlighted here. Thus it is reasonable to theorize that with regard to the GA systems considered in this book, a scale-free network promotes a scale-free dynamics (data illustrated in Figure 1.1).

While this argument suggests that we understand some fundamental features of GA neuronal mechanisms, Sporns warns (p. 274) that "the relation between structural connection patterns and dynamic diversity is far from understood."

Physicist Guido Caldarelli, from the University of Rome Sapienza, has addressed scale-free networks (2007). Pioneered by Herbert Stanley at Boston University, the study of scale-free phenomena has extended to many fields, e.g., percolation (as in a coffeemaker). Mathematicians have discovered such phenomena to have universal properties, including the criticality (sensitive responsivity to small stimuli) associated with phase transitions. When tracking behavior through time, scale-free dynamics yield power law graphs derived from the exponential equations sketched in Chapter 1 and Equation 10.1. Caldarelli and Barabasi's work in this area suggests that a scale-free network can in principle lead to scale-free temporal behavior, although this result is not logically or mathematically guaranteed.

There are at least two points in this discussion to think about. First, regarding Buszaki's and others' arguments about scale-free networks, I have not been able to understand what inferences are rigorously proven as compared to those which are reasonable and attractive speculations.

Secondly, regarding any implications of scale-free systems for regulating GA, it is not necessary that a mathematically pure, exponentially described system exist among the reticular neurons that I discuss. Instead, I emphasize that with a scaling-like network (Figure 6.1), including many low-connected and a few highly connected neurons, the latter deliver an identical, uniform signal which achieves what neuroscientists mean by *integration*. After initiating a GA increase with an NGC signal to many CNS levels, the subsequent well-integrated activities in many neuronal groups are not identical to each other. By analogy to an American football team, the 11 players during an offensive maneuver are not doing the same thing, but they are rigidly following the same overall, coordinated plan. Likewise, the NGC signal and other reticular signals, carried far and wide, initiate activities which are not identical but are still coordinated.

The lessons to take away from network theory include, first, the idea that our A/P, L GA system achieves a consistency of signaling, sending the very same message to the local cellular neighborhood and to far distant neural regions, which is one form of integration. Second, a scale-free GA system has sensitivity and criticality, but is susceptible to severe malfunction if enough nodes such as NGC neurons are damaged.

It has been claimed that scale-free networks with just one major hub may be susceptible to epidemics if that hub is damaged, and thus such networks would be unstable. This concern may not apply in full force to the mammalian brain. In the GA mechanisms reviewed here, medullary NGC certainly comprise a major hub, but giant pontine reticular neurons also contribute. And, for example, Marshall Devor's lab (Minert et al., 2017) have reported a mesopontine tegmental region whose neurons are essential for maintenance of consciousness loss during anesthesia. Having three or more hubs in GA systems may provide for a sufficient level of stability.

A caution about overplaying the applicability of network theory to the brain: such attempts have been going on for a long time. For example, Frank Rosenblatt's "Perceptron" was developed at Cornell during the late 1950s, and Michael Dertouzos used "finite state automata" at MIT during the 1960s. Such developments and similar efforts did little to advance the field of neuroscience. Even now, machine learning proceeds with pseudo-neural nets that achieve their results by routes which remain obscure. I call these nets "pseudo-neural" because the chance that there are important similarities to known neurobiological mechanisms would seem to be very small. Most important, network theorists tend to think in digital languages. Even though, in the brain, we do have "digital" action potentials, there are many other types of mechanisms which constitute "analogue" signaling: dendrite to dendrite, analogue chemical neurotransmitter, and neuropeptide actions *outside* the active synaptic zone of an axon terminal, as well as inside the conventional active synaptic zone. For all of these reasons, it seems wise to think of network theory as a source of ideas for the neuroscientist but nothing more than that.

Fifth, in all important respects, CNS arousal taken from the bottom up is bilaterally symmetric. Unilateral damage will not make the system fall apart because the undamaged side of the GA system functions still sufficiently well.

Sixth, it is possible to resolve differences of opinion among laboratories about the relative importance for GA regulation of different components of ascending arousal pathways. The "low road" comprises signals traveling to and through the hypothalamus, with some axons reaching the large cholinergic neurons of the basal forebrain. As conceived in this book, the hypothalamic signaling path includes unique endocrine links – regulation of stress and sex hormones which govern the *states* of the internal bodily organs as well as instinctive behaviors. Especially in lower animals (but in humans as well) arousal signals through the low-road vertically integrate with body state. From a molecular point of view, hypothalamic hypocretin neurons, all by themselves, serve to illustrate this point.

In contrast, it appears that the "high road," through central thalamus to cerebral cortex, achieves its greatest importance in the human brain. This signaling system supports attention and guided movement through its activation of what Schiff and his colleagues have called a "mesocircuit."

Seventh, the properties of GA suggest rough analogies to developments in the history of mathematical approaches to information and communication science. More than 50 years ago, prominent mathematicians were pioneering work on the cognitive capacities of computers and other electronic devices. In the most elegant development, Claude Shannon (1948) at Bell Labs came up with a simple equation using logarithms to the base 2 (Equation 10.2) to summarize the amount of digital information flow in a series of events (1 to n), (**H**), *without any reference to the specific content or meaning of the message.* In the context of this book, GA is the most prominent term in Equation 1.1 that accounts for the initiation of behavior *without any reference to the specific motivation connected with the behavior.*

$$H = -\sum_{i=1}^{n} P_i (\log P_i)$$

(10.2)

where there is a minus sign because the log of a fractional probability p is negative.

Likewise, the Hungarian-American mathematician John von Neumann (1942, 1948) working at Princeton's Institute for Advanced Study, envisioned the *negative entropy* required for the proper organization of a computing machine. More than 50 years later physicist Jayanth Banavar and I (2007) theoretically proposed *a decrease in chaos* in arousal systems as they go through a phase transition from disordered non-linear firing patterns in the non-aroused state to ordered movement control dynamics (Equation 10.2).

Eighth, Chapter 5 reported data (Figure 5.1 and Equation 5.1) which quantitatively describes the rise of GA as the mouse goes from very low GA (during the light part of the daily cycle) to very high GA (just after the lights go out). Now we can compare that answer to arousal and activity elicited in a different way, by imposing elevated hunger. LeSauter et al. (2009) used wheel running in a mouse experiment during which the time of feeding was restricted and also was advanced into a period in which the mice are usually inactive. The hunger-induced activity, "food anticipatory activity" plotted cumulatively, closely matched a Gaussian function (see Equation 10.3; also called, normal distribution or bell curve), indicating that during each small-time interval the choice between moving and not moving is independent of what happened during the previous interval. Because the binomial distribution of yes–no choices of a discrete random variable approximates – with large Ns of choices – the Gaussian, we note that the results are consistent with the formulation that the mechanisms underlying these behavioral data include a large number of individual, independent neuronal "go/no-go" decisions with an increasing proportion of "go" decisions as feeding time draws near.

$$f = \frac{1}{\sqrt{2\pi\sigma^2}} e^{-\frac{(x-u)^2}{2\sigma^2}} \tag{10.3}$$

where μ is the mean of the distribution, σ is the standard deviation, and σ^2 is the variance.

This summary of an animal brought to high arousal by hunger shows different dynamics from those of an animal brought to high arousal by the change from light to dark (Equation 5.1). Therefore, the point would be that the quantitative signature of the transition from low to high arousal may depend on the environmental cause of the transition.

Ninth, I suspect that all these points apply universally among vertebrates. Fish brain neurophysiologist Donald Faber and I (2012) proposed that NGC neuronal populations comprise an expansion of the fish brain's Mauthner cells. These are huge reticulospinal cells which primarily are essential for rapid escape responses. More generally, it is said by molecular-trained developmental biologists that mechanisms used early in development are more conserved during evolution (e.g., from lab animals to humans) than mechanisms used late in development. Compared to the cerebral cortex, for example, NGC cells in the medulla certainly depend on early developing mechanisms and therefore, as a result, would be expected to be conserved.

Tenth, Chapter 7 sampled high GA behaviors, aggression, sex, and fear. Aggression and sex behaviors, in themselves, require high GA. All these three types of high GA behaviors involve autonomic arousal. Regarding aggression, pharmacological evidence reveals roles for high GA. In particular, a scale-free GA system would enable accelerated acts of aggression, offensive or defensive, as necessary. With regard to fear, evidence from James McGaugh's lab showed clearly that arousal neurotransmitters potentiated fear learning. For sex, of course, hormonal effects on arousal enhance reproductive behaviors in both sexes. Beyond those effects both pharmacological evidence and a GA-breeding program forced the conclusion that high GA, as expected, fosters successful reproductive behaviors.

Eleventh, it is possible to see how the loss of key features of GA systems causes the absence of behavioral activity. Traumatic brain injury interrupts and deep anesthesia severely reduces A/P, L and high connectivity, and so the identity of messages traveling long distances over long axoned neurons is lost.

Some Major Unanswered Questions

1. NGC developmental patterning: what sequences of transcription factors are responsible for deriving different kinds of NGC neurons during embryonic life?
2. How do the longest axon A/P GA axons find their way?
3. Above I refer to the transcriptome discovered in my lab, the mRNAs expressed by NGC neurons which have axonal projections to the thalamus (Tabansky et al., 2018). Unique was their expression of endothelial nitric oxide synthase (eNOS). What about the transcriptomes of other large reticular neurons?
4. The manners in which glutamatergic, glycinergic, and GABAergic neurons in the brainstem reticular formation affect each other through short-axoned connections are still obscure. Can optogenetic approaches address this question?
5. How long will it take to discover possible useful *modulations* of individual neuronal "types" in the medullary reticular formation (cf. Capelli et al., 2017)? To follow up Schiff's et al. (2007) demonstration of the importance of central thalamic activity in the human brain, will we be able to enhance inputs to central thalamus?
6. Are some NGC neurons outside the blood–brain barrier?
7. We must consider the question of susceptibility to epidemics of abnormal activity (reviewed, Barabasi, 2009). Among authors there are differences in emphasis. Certainly, if a hub (a node) in a single-hub scale-free network is damaged, bad things are going to happen. The summary of NGC neuroanatomy, physiology, and genomics in Chapter 2 makes it clear that damage to NGC neurons will harm the ability of the animal to initiate behavior of any sort (e.g., Capelli et al., 2017). Lu and Li (2016) "found that the node-based strategies are often more harmful to the network controllability than the edge-based ones, and so are the recalculated strategies than their counterparts." "The Barabási-Albert scale-free model, which has a highly biased structure, proves to be the most vulnerable of the tested model networks." However, Albert et al. (2000) found that "such (scale-free) networks display an unexpected degree of robustness, the ability of their nodes to communicate being unaffected even by unrealistically high failure rates." That error tolerance comes at a high price in that "these networks are extremely vulnerable to attacks (that is, to the selection and removal of a few nodes that play a vital role" in the network. Of course, for me, this means NGC neurons. Along the same lines, Motter (2004), writing about networks like scale-free ones, said that a small attack or failure has the potential to trigger a global cascade, if a critical fraction of the most connected nodes is removed.

8. How does this "bottom-up" approach to CNS arousal systems match up with and complement classical cortico-centric approaches?

9. Are some of the outstanding properties of GA systems linked to each other? As noted, the length of axons in an A/P, L system with synaptic connections at several levels allows for a high degree of connectivity and, because of these large neurons, raises the possibility of a scale-free system. The large NGC neurons with widespread dendrites, lengthy projections, multimodal sensitivity, and high firing rates show us neurons with incredibly large channel capacity for sending an integrated signal in many directions. What would links among such properties have to do with behavioral cognitive processes?

10. Exactly how might problems with GA mechanisms reviewed in this book contribute to obvious GA problems in the clinic, including depression, stuporous states, Alzheimer's ADHD, problems during aging, or sleep disorders?

11. Exactly how might *improved* regulation of GA mechanisms avoid public health problems as regards vigilance (shift work, military, dangerous occupations) and violent behaviors, among others?

12. Might improved understanding of GA mechanisms shed light on the mysterious fatigue states (CFIDS, Fibromyalgia Syndrome, Gulf War Syndrome)?

Wrapping up, I note that the aims of this book have been somewhat more modest than what some neuroscientists attempt. For example, the well-known computational neuroscientist Stanislas Dehaene and his colleagues (2017) asked, in the prestigious *Science* journal, "What is consciousness and could machines have it?" My book does not ask a question as ambitious as that. Instead I have laid out mechanisms which facilitate *getting to* a state of consciousness. By analogy, if Stanislas Dehaene and his colleagues are in the "attic" of the "house of consciousness," then the mechanisms conceptualized and summarized here show the way to stairs out of the basement. For that purpose, this book has sought to embrace and describe neuroanatomical, neurophysiological, and molecular mechanisms in a solid, clear manner.

Bibliography

Adamantidis A., Zhang F., Aravanis A. M., Deisseroth K., and de Lecea L. (2007). Neural substrates of awakening probed with optogenetic control of hypocretin neurons. *Nature.* 450: 420–5.

Adams J., Graham, D., Jennett, B. (2000). The neuropathology of the vegetative state after an acute brain insult. *Brain.* 123: 1327–38.

Adams Z. M., Forgacs P. B., Conte M. M., Nauvel T. J., Drover J. D. (2016). Late and progressive alterations of sleep dynamics following central thalamic deep brain stimulation (CT-DBS) in chronic minimally conscious state. *Clin Neurophysiol.* 127(9): 3086–92.

Agmo A., Villalpando A. (1995). Central nervous stimulants facilitate sexual behavior in male rats with medial prefrontal cortex lesions. *Brain Res.* 696(1–2):187–93.

Albers H. E. (2015). Species, sex and individual differences in the vasotocin/vasopressin system: relationship to neurochemical signaling in the social behavior neural network. *Front Neuroendocrinol.* 36: 49–71.

Albert R., Jeong H., Barabasi A. L. (2000). Error and attack tolerance of complex networks. *Nature.* 406(6794): 378–82.

Albert F. W., Carlborg O., Plyusnina I., et al. (2009). Genetic architecture of tameness in a rat model of animal domestication. *Genetics.* 182(2): 541–54. doi: 10.1534/genetics.109.102186. Epub 2009 Apr 10.

Allaway K. C., Machold R. (2017). Developmental specification of forebrain cholinergic neurons. *Dev Biol.* 421(1): 1–7.

Alonso L. M., et al. (2014). Dynamical criticality during induction of anesthesia in human ECoG recordings. *Front Neural Circuits.* 8:20. https://doi.org/10.3389/fncir.2014.00020.

Alvarez-Dieppa A. C., et al. (2016). Vagus nerve stimulation enhances extinction of conditioned fear in rats and modulates arc protein, CaMKII, and GluN2B-containing NMDA receptors in the basolateral amygdala. *Neural Plast.* 2016:4273280.

Amaral D. (2000). In *Principles of Neural Science* (4th edition). New York, NY: McGraw-Hill, pp. 331–53.

Anaclet C., Parmentier R., et al. (2009). Orexin/hypocretin and histamine: distinct roles in the control of wakefulness demonstrated using knock-out mouse models. *J Neurosci.* 29(46): 14423–38.

Anderson D. J. (2016). Circuit modules linking internal states and social behaviour in flies and mice. *Nat Rev Neurosci.* 17(11): 692–704.

Andrews-Hanna J. R., et al. (2007). Disruption of large-scale brain systems in advanced aging. *Neuron.* 56(5): 924–35.

Anholt R. R. (2004). Genetic modules and networks for behavior: lessons from *Drosophila. Bioessays.* 26(12): 1299–306.

Antony A. K., Kong W., Lorenz H. P. (2010). Upregulation of neurodevelopmental genes during scarless healing. *Ann Plast Surg.* 64(2): 247–50.

Anthony T. E., et al. (2014). Control of stress-induced persistent anxiety by an extra-amygdala septohypothalamic circuit. *Cell.* 156: 522–36.

Archer J. (1977). Testosterone and persistence in mice. *Anim Behav.* 25(2): 479–88.

Arrieta-Cruz I., Pfaff D. W., Shelley D. N. (2007). Mouse model of diffuse brain damage following anoxia, evaluated by assay of generalized arousal. *Exp Neurol.* 205(2): 449–60.

Aston-Jones G., Cohen J. D. (2005). An integrative theory of locus coeruleus-norepinephrine function: adaptive gain and optimal performance. *Ann Rev Neurosci.* 28: 403–50.

Aston-Jones G., Zhu Y., Card J. P. (2004). Numerous GABAergic afferents to locus ceruleus in the pericerulear dendritic zone: possible interneuronal pool. *J Neurosci.* 24(9): 2313–21.

Aston-Jones G., et al. (1996). Role of the locus coeruleus in emotional activation. *Prog Brain Res.* 107: 379–402.

Aston-Jones G., et al. (2001). A neural circuit for circadian regulation of arousal. *Nat Neurosci.* 4: 732–8.

Autret A., Lucas B., Mondon K., et al. (2001). Sleep and brain lesions: a critical review of the literature and additional new cases. *Neurophysiol Clin.* 31: 356–75.

Azevedo R. T., Badoud D., Tsakiris M. (2017). Afferent cardiac signals modulate attentional engagement to low spatial frequency fearful faces. *Cortex.* pii: S0010-9452(17)30205-8.

Azmitia E. (2010). Evolution of serotonin: sunlight to suicide. In: Muller C., Jacobs B. (Eds.), *Handbook of Behavioral Neurobiology of Serotonin.* San Diego, CA: Elsevier/Academic Press, pp. 125–61.

Bai Y. J., et al. (2009). Orexin A attenuates unconditioned sexual motivation in male rats. *Pharmacol Biochem Behav.* 91(4): 581–9.

Baker J. L., et al. (2016). Robust modulation of arousal regulation, performance, and frontostriatal activity through central thalamic deep brain stimulation in healthy nonhuman primates. *J Neurophysiol.* 116(5): 2383–404.

Barabási A. L. (2009). Scale-free networks: a decade and beyond. *Science.* 325: 412–13.

Barabasi A. L. (2002). *Linked: The New Science of Networks.* Cambridge, MA: Perseus.

Barabasi A.-L. (2015). Spectrum of controlling and observing complex networks. *Nat Phys.* 11: 779–96.

Barabasi A. L., Albert R. (1999). Emergence of scaling in random networks. *Science.* 286(5439): 509–12.

Barabási A. L. et al. (2011). Network medicine: a network-based approach to human disease. *Nat Rev Genet.* 12(1): 56–68.

Bargiello T. A., Young M. W. (1984). Molecular genetics of a biological clock in *Drosophila. Proc Natl Acad Sci U S A.* 81(7): 2142–6.

Barrett L. F. (2017). *How Emotions Are Made.* Boston, MA: Houghton Mifflin Harcourt.

Bartolomeo P., Chokron S. (2002). Orienting of attention in left unilateral neglect. *Neurosci Biobehav Rev.* 26(2): 217–34.

Barzel B., Liu Y., Barabasi A.-L. (2015). Constructing minimal models for complex system dynamics. *Nat Commun.* 6: 1–8.

Bass J., Lazar M. A. (2016). Circadian time signatures of fitness and disease. *Science.* 354: 994–9.

Bassett D. S., et al. (2006). Adaptive reconfiguration of fractal small world human brain functional networks. *PNAS.* 103: 19518–23.

Bassett D. S., Sporns O. (2017) Article I. Network nueroscience. *Nat Neurosci.* 20(3): 353–64. doi: 10.1038/nn.4502.

Bassetti C. L. (2011). Sleep and stroke. In: Kryger M. H., Roth T., Dement W. C. (Eds.), *Principles and Practice of Sleep Medicine,* 5th edn. Philadelphia, PA: Saunders, pp. 993–1015.

Batini C., Moruzzi G., Palestini M., Rossi G. F., Zanchetti A. (1959). Effects of complete pontine transections on the sleep-wakefulness rhythm: the midpontine pretri-geminal preparation. *Arch Ital Biol.* 97: 1–12.

Becker J., et al. (Eds.). (2008). *Sex Differences in the Brain.* New York, NY: Oxford University Press.

Beckstead R. M., Domesick V. B., Nauta W. J. (1979). Efferent connections of the substantia nigra and ventral tegmental area in the rat. *Brain Res.* 175: 191–217.

Bedrosian T. A., Nelson R. J. (2014). Nitric oxide and serotonin interactions in aggression. *Curr Top Behav Neurosci.* 17: 131–42.

Behn C., Brown E., Scammell T., Kopell N. (2007). Mathematical model of network dynamics governing mouse sleep-wake behavior. *J Neurophysiol.* 97:382803840.

Beitz A. J. (1982). The organization of afferent projections to the midbrain periaqueductal gray of the rat. *Neuroscience.* 7(1): 133–59.

Benarroch E. E. (2013). Pedunculopontine nucleus: functional organization and clinical implications. *Neurology.* 80(12): 1148–55.

Beretzner F., Brownstone R. M. (2013). Lhx3–Chx10 reticulospinal neurons in locomotor circuits. *J Neurosci.* 33: 14681–92.

Berntson G. G., Shafi R., Sarter M. (2002). Specific contributions of the basal forebrain corticopetal cholinergic system to electroencephalographic activity and sleep/waking behaviour. *Eur J Neurosci.* 16: 2453–61.

Berridge C. W. (2008). Noradrenergic modulation of arousal. *Brain Res Rev.* 58: 1–17.

Berridge, C. W., Foote S. L. (1991). Effects of locus coeruleus activation on EEG activity in neocortex and hippocampus. *J Neurosci.* 11: 3135–45.

(1996). Enhancement of behavioral and electroencephalographic indices of waking following stimulation of noradrenergic beta-receptors within the medial septal region of the basal forebrain. *J Neurosci.* 16: 6999–7009.

Berridge C. W., Waterhouse B. D. (2003). The locus coeruleus-noradrenergic system: modulation of behavioral state and state-dependent cognitive processes. *Brain Res Rev.* 42: 33–84.

Bharos T. B., Kuypers H. G., Lemon R. N., Muir R. B. (1981). Divergent collaterals from deep cerebellar neurons to thalamus and tectum, and to medulla oblongata and spinal cord: retrograde fluorescent and electrophysiological studies. *Exp Brain Res.* 42(3-4):399–410.

Blair R.J., Peschardt K.S., Budhani S., Mitchell D.G., Pine D.S. (2006). Article I. The development of psychopathy. *J Child Psychol Psychiatry.* 47(3-4):262–76.

Blanco-Centurion C., Xu MC., Murillo-Rodriguez E., et al. (2006). Adenosine and sleep homeostasis in the basal forebrain. *J Neurosci.* 26: 8092–100.

Blanco-Centurion C., Gerashchenko D., Shiromani P. J. (2007). Effects of saporin-induced lesions of three arousal populations on daily levels of sleep and wake. *J Neurosci.* 27(51): 14041–8.

Blaustein J. D., Turcotte J. C. (1989). Estradiol-induced progestin receptor immunoreactivity is found only in estrogen receptor-immunoreactive cells in guinea pig brain. *Neuroendocrinology.* 49(5): 454–61.

Block, N. (2007). *Consciousness, Function and Representation.* Cambridge, MA: MIT Press.

Blumbergs P. C., Jones N. R., North J. B. (1989). Diffuse axonal injury in head trauma. *J Neurol Neurosurg Psychiatry.* 52: 838–41.

Blumenfeld H., McCormick D. A. (2000). Corticothalamic inputs control the pattern of activity generated in thalamocortical networks. *J Neurosci.* 20(13): 5153–62.

Bodart O., et al. (2017). Measures of metabolism and complexity in the brain of patients with disorders of consciousness. *Neuroimage Clin.* 14: 354–62.

Bonnelle, V., et al. (2012). Salience network integrity predicts default mode network function after traumatic brain injury. *PNAS.* 109: 4690–5.

Borbely A. A. (1982). A two process model of sleep regulation. *Human Neurobiol.* 1: 195–204.

Borbely A. A., Tobler I. (1985). Homeostatic and circadian principles in sleep regulation in the rat. In: McGinty D. J., et al. (Eds.), *Brain Mechanisms of Sleep.* New York, NY: Raven Press, pp. 35–44.

Boutrel B., Cannella N., de Lecea L. (2010). The role of hypocretin in driving arousal and goal-oriented behaviors. *Brain Res.* 1324: 103–11.

Bremer F. (1935). Cerveau isole et physiologie du sommeil. *CR Soc Biol (Paris).* 118: 1235–42.

Brink E. E., Pfaff D. W. (1981). Supraspinal and segmental input to lumbar epaxial motoneurons in the rat. *Brain Res.* 226: 43–60.

Broadbent D. E. (1971). *Decision and Stress.* London: Academic Press.

Brookes M. J., et al. (2011). Investigating the electrophysiological basis of resting state networks using magnetoencephalography. *PNAS.* 108: 16783–8.

Broom L., et al. (2017). A translational approach to capture gait signatures of neurological disorders in mice and humans. *Sci Rep.* 7(1): 3225. doi: 10.1038/s41598-017-03336-1.

Brown R. E., McKenna J. T. (2015). Turning a negative into a positive: ascending GABAergic control of cortical activation and arousal. *Front Neurol.* 6:135. doi: 10.3389/fneur.2015.00135.

Brown R. E., et al. (2006). Electrophysiological characterization of neurons in the dorsolateral pontine rapid-eye-movement sleep induction zone of the rat: intrinsic membrane properties and responses to carbachol and orexins. *Neuroscience.* 143(3): 739–55.

Brown E. N., Lydic R., Schiff N. D. (2010). General anesthesia, sleep, and coma. *New Engl J Med.* 363(27): 2638–50.

Brust J., (2000). In *Principles of Neural Science* (4th edition). New York, NY: McGraw-Hill, pp. 1302–16.

Buchanan G., Richerson G. (2010). Central serotonin neurons are required for arousal to CO_2. *Proc Natl Acad Sci.* 107: 16354–9.

Buckner R. L., et al. (2008). The brain's default network anatomy, function, and relevance to disease. *Ann NY Acad Sci.* 1124: 1–38.
(2009). Cortical hubs revealed by intrinsic functional connectivity: mapping, assessment of stability, and relation to Alzheimer's disease. *J Neurosci.* 29(6): 1860–73.
(2011). The organization of the human cerebellum estimated by intrinsic functional connectivity. *J Neurophysiol.* 106: 2322–45.

Bullmore E., Sporns O. (2009). Complex brain networks: graph theoretical analysis of structural and functional systems. *Nature Rev Neurosci.* 10(3): 186–98.

Butler M. P., Karatsoreos I. N., LeSauter J., Silver R. (2012). Dose-dependent effects of androgens on the circadian timing system and its response to light. *Endocrinology.* 153(5): 2344–52.

Buzsaki G. (2006). *Rhythms of the Brain.* NewYork, NY: Oxford University Press.

Buzsáki G., Schomburg E. W. (2015). What does gamma coherence tell us about inter-regional neural communication? *Nat Neurosci.* 18(4): 484–9.

Buzsaki G., Bickford R. G., Ponomareff G., et al. (1998). Nucleus basalis and thalamic control of neocortical activity in the freely moving rat. *J Neurosci.* 8: 4007–26.

Buzsáki G., Geisler C., Henze D. A., Wang X. J. (2004). Interneuron diversity series: circuit complexity and axon wiring economy of cortical interneurons. *Trends Neurosci.* 27: 186–93.

Caballero P. E. J. (2010). Bilateral paramedian thalamic artery infarcts: report of 10 cases. *J Stroke Cardiovasc Dis.* 19: 283–9.

Caggiano V., et al. (2017). Midbrain circuits that set locomotor speed and gait selection. *Nature.* 553(7689): 455–60.

Caldarelli G. (2007). *Scale-Free Networks.* Oxford: Oxford University Press.

Calderon D. P., Proekt A., Pfaff D. (2018). Activation of large neurons in the medullary reticular formation regulates cortical and behavioral arousal. *Nat Neurosci.* (submitted).

Calderon D. P., et al. (2016). Generalized CNS arousal: an elementary force within the vertebrate nervous system. *Neurosci Biobehav Rev.* 68: 167–76.

Caldwell H., Albers H. E. (2016). Oxytocin, vasopressin, and the motivational forces that drive social behaviors. *Curr Topics Behav Neurosci.* 27: 51–103.

Cantero J. L., Atienza M. (2005). The role of neural synchronization in the emergence of cognition across the wake-sleep cycle. *Rev Neurosci.* 16(1): 69–83.

Cape E. G., Jones B. E. (2000). Effects of glutamate agonist versus procaine microinjections into the basal forebrain cholinergic cell area upon gamma and theta EEG activity and sleep–wake state. *Eur J Neurosci.* 12(6): 2166–84.

Capelli P., et al. (2017). Locomotor speed control circuits in the caudal brainstem. *Nature.* 551(7680): 373–7.

Carroll M. E., Anker J. J. (2010). Sex differences and ovarian hormones in animal models of drug dependence. *Horm Behav.* 58(1): 44–56.

Carter M. E., Adamantidis A., Ohtsu H., Deisseroth K., de Lecea L. (2009a). Sleep homeostasis modulates hypocretin-mediated sleep-to-wake transitions. *J Neurosci.* 29(35): 10939–49.

Carter M. E., Borg J. S., de Lecea L. (2009b). The brain hypocretins and their receptors: mediators of allostatic arousal. *Curr Opin Pharmacol.* 9(1): 39–45. Review.

Carter M. E., et al. (2010). Tuning arousal with optogenetic modulation of locus coeruleus neurons. *Nat Neurosci.* 13(12): 1526–33.

Carter M. E., Brill J., Bonnavion P., et al. (2012). Mechanism for hypocretin-mediated sleep-to-wake transitions. *Proc Natl Acad Sci U S A.* 109:E2635–44.

Carter M. E., de Lecea L., Adamantidis A. (2013). Functional wiring of hypocretin and LC-NE neurons: implications for arousal. *Front Behav Neurosci.* 20(7): 43.

Casaratto S. (2016). Stratification of unresponsive patients by an independently validated index of brain complexity. *Ann Neurol.* 80: 718–29.

Cedarbaum J. M., Aghajanian G. K. (1978). Afferent projections to the rat locus coeruleus as determined by a retrograde tracing technique. *J Comp Neurol.* 178(1): 1–16.

Cembrowski M. S., et al. (2016). Hipposeq: a comprehensive RNA-seq database of gene expression in hippocampal principal neurons. *Elife.* 5: e14997.

Chamberlin N. L., Saper C. B. (1992). Topographic organization of cardiovascular responses to electrical and glutamate microstimulation of the parabrachial nucleus in the rat. *J Comp Neurol.* 326(2): 245–62.

(1994). Topographic organization of respiratory responses to glutamate microstimulation of the parabrachial nucleus in the rat. *J Neurosci.* 14: 6500–10.

Chandler D. J., Waterhouse B. D., Gao W. J. (2014). New perspectives on catecholaminergic regulation of executive circuits: evidence for independent modulation of prefrontal functions by midbrain dopaminergic and noradrenergic neurons. *Front Neural Circuits.* 8:53. doi: 10.3389/fncir.2014.00053.

Chemelli R., et al. (1999). Narcolepsy in orexin knockout mice: molecular genetic and sleep regulation. *Cell.* 98: 437–51.

Chen J., Randeva H. S. (2004). Genomic organization of mouse orexin receptors. *Mol. Endocrinol.* 18: 2790–804.

Chen C. T., Dun S. L., Kwok E. H., Dun N. J., Chang J. K. (1999). Orexin A-like immunoreactivity in the rat brain. *Neurosci Lett.* 260: 161–4.

Chen C., et al. (2015). Testosterone modulates preattentive sensory processing and involuntary attention switches to emotional voices. *J Neurophysiol.* 113(6): 1842–9.

Chennu S., et al. (2017). Brain networks predict metabolism, diagnosis and prognosis at the bedside in disorders of consciousness. *Brain.* 140: 2120–32.

Chou T. C., Bjorkum A. A., Gaus S. E., et al. (2002). Afferents to the ventrolateral preoptic nucleus. *J Neurosci.* 22: 977–90.

Chou T. C., Scammell T. E., Gooley J. J., et al. (2003). Critical role of dorsomedial hypothalamic nucleus in a wide range of behavioral circadian rhythms. *J Neurosci.* 23(33): 10691–702.

Christensen J. A., et al. (2015). Sleep-stage transitions during polysomnographic recordings as diagnostic features of type 1 narcolepsy. *Sleep Med.* 16(12): 1558–66.

Chung S., et al. (2017). Identification of preoptic sleep neurons using retrograde

labeling and gene profiling. *Nature.* 545: 477–82.

Ciriello J., de Oliveira C. V. R., Masoumeh M., et al. (2002). Estrogen alters the cardiovascular responses to activation of rostral ventrolateral medulla in the female. *Soc Neurosci Abs.* 768:6.

Claassen J., et al. (2013). Recommendations on the use of EEG monitoring in critically ill patients: consensus statement from the neurointensive care section of the ESICM. *Intensive Care Med.* 39(8): 1337–51.

(2016). Bedside quantitative electroencephalography improves assessment of consciousness in comatose subarachnoid hemorrhage patients. *Ann Neurol.* 80(4): 541–53.

Claiborne J. A., Nag S., Mokha S. S. (2009). Article I. Estrogen-dependent, sex-specific modulation of mustard oil-induced secondary thermal hyperalgesia by orphanin FQ in the rat. *Neurosci Lett.* 456(2): 59–63. doi: 10.1016/j.neulet.2009.03.106. Epub 2009 Apr 5.

Clipperton-Allen A. E., et al. (2010). Agonistic behavior in males and females: Effects of an estrogen receptor beta agonist in gonadectomized and gonadally intact mice. *Psychoneuroendocrinology.* 35(7): 1008–22.

Cohen J. E. (1995). Unexpected dominance of high frequencies in chaotic nonlinear population models. *Nature.* 378: 610–16.

Cohen M. S., Schwartz-Giblin S., Pfaff D. W. (1987). Brainstem reticular stimulation facilitates back muscle motoneuronal responses to pudendal nerve input. *Brain Res.* 405: 155–61.

Colvin G. B., Whitmoyer D. I., Lisk R. D. et al. (1968). Changes in sleep-wakefulness in female rats during circadian and estrous cycles. *Brain Res.* 7(2): 173–81.

Colvin G. B., Whitmoyer D. I., Sawyer C. H. (1968). Circadian sleep-wakefulness patterns in rats after ovariectomy and treatment with estrogen. *Exp Neurol.* 25(4): 616–25.

Conrad L. A., Pfaff D. W. (1975). Axonal projections of medial preoptic and anterior hypothalamic neurons. *Science.* 190: 1112–14.

Conrad L., Leonard C., Pfaff D. (1974). Connections of the median and dorsal raphe nuclei in the rat: an autoradiographic and degeneration study. *J Comp Neurol.* 156: 179–205.

Conrad, L. C. A., Pfaff, D. W. (1976a). Efferents from medial basal forebrain and hypothalamus in the rat. I. An autoradiography study of the medial preoptic area. *J. Comp. Neurol.*, 169: 185–220.

(1976b). Efferents from medial basal forebrain and hypothalamus in the rat. II. An autoradiography study of the anterior hypothalamus. *J. Comp. Neurol.*, 169: 221–62.

Cools R., Nakamura K., Daw, N. (2011). Serotonin and dopamine: unifying affective, activational and decision functions. *Neuropsychopharmacology.* 36: 98–113.

Corazzol M., et al. (2017). Restoring consciousness with vagal nerve stimulation. *Curr Biol.* 27, R1–R3, September 25, 2017 © 2017Elsevier Ltd. R1

Cottingham S. L., Femano P. A., Pfaff D. W. (1987). Electrical stimulation of the midbrain central gray facilitates reticulospinal activation of axial muscle EMG. *Exp Neurol.* 97(3): 704–24.

(1988). Vestibulospinal and reticulospinal interactions in the activation of back muscle EMG in the rat. *Exp Brain Res.* 73(1): 198–208.

Courtoy P. J., Boyles J. (1983). Fibronectin in the microvasculature: localization in the pericyte-endothelial interstitium. *J Ultrastruct Res.* 83:258–73.

Crick F., Koch C. (2003). A framework for consciousness. *Nat Neurosci.* 6: 119–29.

Csete M., Doyle J. (2004). Bowties, metabolism and disease. *Trends Biotechnol.* 22: 446–50.

Cullinan, W. E., Zaborszky L. (1991). Organization of ascending hypothalamic projections to the rostral forebrain with special reference to the innervation of cholinergic projection neurons. *J Comp Neurol.* 306: 631–67.

Curtis A. L., Valentino R. J. (1994). Corticotropin-releasing factor neurotransmission in locus coeruleus: a possible site of antidepressant action. *Brain Res Bull.* 35(5–6):581–7.

Curtis A. L., Bello N. T., Connolly K. R., Valentino R. J. (2002). Corticotropin-releasing factor neurones of the central nucleus of the amygdala mediate locus coeruleus activation by cardiovascular stress. *J Neuroendocrinol.* 14(8): 667–82.

Da Silva J. A., et al. (2018). Dopamine neuron activity before initiation gates and invigorates future movements. *Proc Natl Acad Sci.* 554: 244–50.

Danielle S., Bassett B. S., Olaf Sporns O. (2017). Network neuroscience. *Nat Neurosci.* 20: 353–64.

Datta S., Hobson J. A. (1995). Suppression of ponto-geniculo-occipital waves by neurotoxic lesions of pontine caudo-lateral peribrachial cells. *Neuroscience.* 67(3): 703–12.

Datta S., Maclean R. R. (2007). Neurobiological mechanisms for the regulation of mammalian sleep-wake behavior: reinterpretation of historical evidence and inclusion of contemporary cellular and molecular evidence. *Neurosci Biobehav Rev.* 31: 775–824.

Datta S., Siwek D. F. (2002). Single cell activity patterns of pedunculopontine tegmentum neurons across the sleep-wake cycle in the freely moving rats. *J Neurosci Res.* 70: 611–21.

Davidson R., Begley S. (2012). *The Emotional Life of your Brain.* NewYork, NY: Hudson St. Press (Penguin).

Davis G. E., Senger D. R. (2005). Endothelial extracellular matrix: biosynthesis, remodeling, and functions during vascular morphogenesis and neovessel stabilization. *Circ Res.* 97:1093–107.

de Biase S., et al. (2017). Investigational therapies for the treatment of narcolepsy. *Expert Opin Investigat Drugs.* 26(8): 953–63.

Deco G., Hagmann P., Hudetz A. G., Tononi G. (2014). Modeling resting-state functional networks when the cortex falls asleep: local and global changes. *Article IV. Cereb Cortex.* 24(12): 3180–94. doi: 10.1093/cercor/bht176. Epub 2013 Jul 10.

de Falco F. A, et al. (1994). Bilateral thalamic damage, cortical hypometabolism and behavioural disturbances. *Eur J Neurol.* 1(2): 165–9.

de Lecea L., Kilduff T.S., Peyron C., et al. (1998). The hypocretins: hypothalamus-specific peptides with neuroexcitatory activity. *Proc. Natl Acad Sci.* 95: 322–7.

Dehaene S., Christen Y. (2011). *Characterizing Consciousness: From Cognition to the Clinic?* Heidelberg: Fondation IPSEN, pp. 55–83.

Dehaene S., et al. (2001a). Cerebral mechanisms of word masking and unconscious repetition priming. *Nat Neurosci.* 4: 752–8.

(2001b). Toward a cognitive neuroscience of consciousness. *Cognition.* 79: 1–37.

Dehaene S., Lau H., Kouider S. (2017). What is consciousness and could machines have it? *Science.* 358: 486–92.

Del Negro C. A., Funk G. D., Feldman J. L. (2018). Breathing matters. *Nat Rev Neurosci.* 19(6): 351–367.

DeLuca D. S., Levin J. Z., Sivachenko A., et al. (2012). RNA-SeQC: RNA-seq metrics for quality control and process optimization. *Bioinformatics.* 28, 1530–2.

Demertzi A., et al. (2015). Intrinsic functional connectivity differentiates minimally conscious from unresponsive patients. *Brain.* 138(Pt 9):2619–31.

Dempsey E. W., Morison R. S. (1942a). The production of rhythmically recurrent cortical potentials after localized thalamic stimulation. *Am J Physiol.* 135: 293–300.

(1942b). The interaction of certain spontaneous and induced cortical potentials. *Am J Physiol.* 135: 301–8.

Dennett D. C. (1991). *Consciousness Explained.* Boston, MA: Little Brown.

Denno D. W. (1990). *Biology and Violence, from Birth to Adulthood.* Cambridge: Cambridge University Press.

Denoyer M., Sallanon M., Buda C., Kitahama K., Jouvet M. (1991). Neurotoxic lesion of the mesencephalic reticular formation and/or the posterior hypothalamus does not alter waking in the cat. *Brain Res.* 539: 287–303.

Deurveilher S., Semba K. (2004). Indirect projections from the suprachiasmatic nucleus to major arousal-promoting cell groups in rat: implications for the circadian control of behavioral state. *Neuroscience.* 130: 165–84.

Devi L., Fricker L. (2016a). Transmitters and peptides: basic principles. In: Pfaff D. W., Volkow N. D. (Eds.), *Neuroscience in the 21st Century* (2nd edition, volume 3). New York, NY: Springer Verlag, pp. 1746–62.

(2016b). Transmitter and peptide receptors: basic principles. In: Pfaff D. W., Volkow, N. D. (Eds.), *Neuroscience in the 21st Century* (2nd edition, volume 3). New York, NY: Springer Verlag, pp. 1763–86.

Devidze N., et al. (2008). Presynaptic actions of opioid receptor agonists in ventromedial hypothalamic neurons in estrogen-and oil-treated female mice. *Neuroscience.* 152(4): 942–9.

(2010). Estradiol regulation of lipocalin-type prostaglandin D synthase promoter activity: evidence for direct and indirect mechanisms. *Neuroscience Lett.* 474(1): 17–21.

Dietrich T., et al. (2001). Effects of blood estrogen level on cortical activation patterns during cognitive activation as measured by functional MRI. *Neuroimage.* 13(3): 425–32.

Dijk D.J., Winsky-Sommerer R. (2016). Sleep and dreamless mice. *Nature.* 539: 364–5.

Dina O. A., et al. (2001). Sex hormones regulate the contribution of PKCepsilon and PKA signalling in inflammatory pain in the rat. *Eur J Neurosci.* 13(12): 2227–33.

Divac I., Björklund A., Lindvall O., Passingham R. E. (1978). Converging projections from the mediodorsal thalamic nucleus and mesencephalic dopaminergic neurons to the neocortex in three species. *J Comp Neurol.* 180(1): 59–71.

Dobin A., Davis C. A., Schlesinger F., et al. (2013). STAR: ultrafast universal RNA-seq aligner. *Bioinformatics.* 29:15–21.

Doesburg S. M., Roggeveen A. B., Kitajo K., Ward L. M. (2008). Large-scale gamma-band phase synchronization and selective attention. *Cerebr Cortex.* 18(2): 386–96.

Dordea A. C., et al. (2016). Androgen-sensitive hypertension associated with soluble guanylate cyclase-α1 deficiency is mediated by 20-HETE. *Am J Physiol Heart Circ Physiol.* 310(11):H1790–800.

Doria V. et al. (2010). Emergence of resting state networks in the preterm human brain. *PNAS.* 107: 20015–20.

Doyle J., Csete M. (2005). Motifs, stability and control. *PLoS Biol.* 3:e392.

Drew T., Rossignol S. (1990a). Functional organization within the medullary reticular formation of intact unanesthetized cat. I. Movements evoked by microstimulation. *J Neurophysiol.* 64(3): 767–81.

(1990b). Functional organization within the medullary reticular formation of intact unanesthetized cat. II. Electromyographic activity evoked by microstimulation. *J Neurophysiol*. 64(3): 782–95.

Drew T., Dubuc R., Rossignol S. (1986). Discharge patterns of reticulospinal and other reticular neurons in chronic, unrestrained cats walking on a treadmill. *J Neurophysiol*. 55(2): 375–401.

Dringenberg H. C., Olmstead M. C. (2003). Integrated contributions of basal forebrain and thalamus to neocortical activation elicited by pedunculopontine tegmental stimulation in urethane-anesthetized rats. *Neuroscience*. 119: 839–53.

Drover J. D., Schiff N. D., Victor J. D. (2010). Dynamics of coupled thalamocortical modules. *J. Comput Neurosci*. 28: 605–16.

Duffy E. (1962). *Activation and Behavior*. New York, NY: Wiley.

Dupré C., et al. (2010). Histaminergic responses by hypothalamic neurons that regulate lordosis and their modulation by estradiol. *Proc Natl Acad Sci U S A*. 107(27): 12311–6.

Easton A., Dwyer E., Pfaff D. W. (2006). Estradiol and orexin-2 saporin actions on multiple forms of behavioral arousal in female mice. *Behav Neurosci*. 120(1): 1–9.

Eberhart J. A., Morrell J. I., Krieger M. S., Pfaff D. W. (1985). An autoradiographic study of projections ascending from the midbrain central gray, and from the region lateral to it, in the rat. *J Comp Neurol*. 241(3): 285–310.

Edlow B. L., et al. (2017). Early detection of consciousness in patients with acute severe traumatic brain injury. *Brain*. 140(9): 2399–414.

Edwards S. B., de Olmos J. S. (1976). Autoradiographic studies of the projections of the midbrain reticular formation: ascending projections of nucleus cuneiformis. *J Comp Neurol*. 165(4): 417–31.

Ekstrand M. I., Nectow A. R., Knight Z. A., et al. (2014). Molecular profiling of neurons based on connectivity. *Cell*. 157, 1230–42.

Elam M., Svensson T. H., Thoren P. (1985). Differentiated cardiovascular afferent regulation of locus coeruleus neurons and sympathetic nerves. *Brain Res*. 358(1–2):77–84.

Elam M., Thorén P., Svensson T. H. (1986). Locus coeruleus neurons and sympathetic nerves: activation by visceral afferents. *Brain Res*. 375(1): 117–25.

Elam M., Yao T., Svensson T. H., Thoren P. (1984). Regulation of locus coeruleus neurons and splanchnic, sympathetic nerves by cardiovascular afferents. *Brain Res*. 290(2): 281–7.

Elisevich K. V., Hrycyshyn A. W., Flumerfelt B. A. (1985). Cerebellar, medullary and spinal afferent connections of the paramedian reticular nucleus in the cat. *Brain Res*. 332(2): 267–82.

Elmquist J. K., et al. (1997). Leptin activates neurons in ventrobasal hypothalamus and brainstem. *Endocrinology*. 138(2): 839–42.

Ericson H., Blomqvist A. (1988). Tracing of neuronal connections with cholera toxin subunit B: light and electron microscopic immunohistochemistry using monoclonal antibodies. *J Neurosci Meth*. 24: 225–35.

España R. A., Reis K. M., Valentino R. J., Berridge C. W. (2005). Organization of hypocretin/orexin efferents to locus coeruleus and basal forebrain arousal-related structures. *J Comp Neurol*. 481(2): 160–78.

Evans S. M., Foltin R. W. (2010). Does the response to cocaine differ as a function of sex or hormonal status in human and non-human primates? *Horm Behav*. 58(1): 13–21.

Eysenck H. J., Eysenck S. B. (1967). On the unitary nature of extraversion. *Acta Psychol (Amst)*. 26(4): 383–90.

Faber D. S., et al. (1989). Neuronal networks underlying the escape response in goldfish. *Ann N Y Acad Sci*. 563: 11–33.

Fadok J. P., et al. (2017). A competitive inhibitory circuit for selection of active and passive fear responses. *Nature*. 542: 96–105.

Fantin A., Maden C. H., Ruhrberg C. (2009). Neuropilin ligands in vascular and neuronal patterning. *Biochem Soc Trans*. 37(Pt 6): 1228–32.

Fardin V., Oliveras J. L., Besson J. M. (1984). Projections from the periaqueductal gray matter to the B3 cellular area (nucleus raphe magnus and nucleus reticularis paragigantocellularis) as revealed by the retrograde transport of horseradish peroxidase in the rat. *J Comp Neurol.* 223(4): 483–500.

Feliers D., Chen X., Akis N., et al. (2005). VEGF regulation of endothelial nitric oxide synthase in glomerular endothelial cells. *Kidney Int.* 68:1648–59.

Fetcho J. R., McLean D. L. (2010). Some principles of organization of spinal neurons underlying locomotion in zebrafish and their implications. *Annals N Y Acad Sci.* 1198: 94–104.

Filosa J. A., Iddings J. A. (2013). Astrocyte regulation of cerebral vascular tone. *Am J Physiol Heart Circ Physiol.* 305:H609–619.

Fins J. J. (2015). *Brain Comes to Mind.* Cambridge: Cambridge University Press.

Fiset P., et al. (1999). Brain mechanisms of propofol-induced loss of consciousness in humans: a positron emission tomographic study. *J Neurosci.* 19(13): 5506–13.

Flavell S. W., et al. (2013). Serotonin and the neuropeptide PDF initiate and extend opposing behavioral states in *C. elegans*. *Cell.* 154(5): 1023–35.

Fogerson P. M., Huguenard J. R. (2016). Tapping the brakes: cellular and synaptic mechanisms that regulate thalamic oscillations. *Neuron.* 92(4): 687–704.

Fontani G., et al. (2004). Attentional, emotional and hormonal data in subjects of different ages. *Eur J Appl Physiol.* 92: 452–61.

Forgacs P. B., et al. (2017). Dynamic regimes of neocortical activity linked to corticothalamic integrity correlate with outcomes in acute anoxic brain injury after cardiac arrest. *Ann Clin Transl Neurol.* 4(2): 119–29.

Fornito A., et al. (2012). Competitive and cooperative dynamics of large-scale brain functional networks supporting recollection. *PNAS.* 109: 12788–93.

Fox M. D., et al. (2005). The human brain is intrinsically organized into dynamic anticorrelated functional networks. *PNAS.* 102: 9673–8.
(2006). Spontaneous neuronal activity distinguishes human dorsal and ventral attention systems. *PNAS.* 103: 10046–51.

Fregosi M., et al. (2017). Corticobulbar projections from distinct motor cortical areas to the reticular formation in macaque monkeys. *Eur J Neurosci.* doi: 10.1111/ejn.13576.

Fridman E. A., et al. (2014). Regional cerebral metabolic patterns demonstrate the role of anterior forebrain mesocircuit dysfunction in the severely injured brain. *Proc Natl Acad Sci U S A.* 111(17): 6473–8.

Frohlich J., et al. (2001). Statistical analysis of measures of arousal in ovariectomized female mice. *Horm Behav.* 39(1): 39–47. (2002). Statistical analysis of hormonal influences on arousal measures in ovariectomized female mice. *Horm Behav.* 2(4): 414–23.

Frohmader K. S., Pitchers K. K., Balfour M. E., Coolen L. M. (2010). Mixing pleasures: review of the effects of drugs on sex behavior in humans and animal models. *Horm Behav.* 58(1): 149–62.

Fuller P. M., Gooley J. J., Saper C. B. (2006). Neurobiology of the sleep–wake cycle: sleep architecture, circadian regulation, and regulatory feedback. *J Biol Rhythms.* 21: 482–93.

Fuller P. M., Saper C. B., Lu J. (2007). The pontine REM switch: past and present. *J Physiol.* 584: 735–41.

Fuller P. M., et al. (2011). Reassessment of the structural basis of the ascending arousal system. *J Comp Neurol.* 519(5): 933–56.

Fulwiler C. E., Saper C. B. (1984). Subnuclear organization of the efferent connections of the parabrachial nucleus in the rat. *Brain Res.* 319: 229–59.

Funato H., et al. (2016). Forward-genetics analysis of sleep in randomly mutagenized mice. *Nature.* 539: 378–87.

Gagnidze K., Weil Z., Khattak M., Pfaff D. (2010). Estrogen-induced chromatin remodeling and gene transcription in ventromedial hypothalamus. *Soc Neurosci.* Abstract #495.11 (Poster)

Gallager D. W., Pert A. (1978). Afferents to brain stem nuclei (brain stem raphe, nucleus reticularis pontis caudalis and nucleus gigantocellularis) in the rat as demonstrated by microiontophoretically applied horseradish peroxidase. *Brain Res.* 144(2): 257–75.

Gao J., Barzel B., Barabasi A.-L. (2016). Universal resilience patterns in complex systems. *Nature.* 530: 307–12.

Garcia-Cardena G., Fan R., Shah V., et al. (1998). Dynamic activation of endothelial nitric oxide synthase by Hsp90. *Nature.* 392:821–4.

Garcia-Rill E., Skinner R. D., Gilmore S. A., Owings R. (1983). Connections of the mesencephalic locomotor region (MLR) II. Afferents and efferents. *Brain Res Bull.* 10(1): 63–71.

Garcia-Rill E. (2015a). The physiology of the pedunculopontine nucleus: implications for deep brain stimulation. *J Neural Transm (Vienna).* 122(2): 225–35.
(2015b). *Waking and the Reticular Activating System in Health and Disease.* San Diego, CA: Academic Press/Elsevier.

Garel S., López-Bendito G. (2014). Inputs from the thalamocortical system on axon pathfinding mechanisms. *Curr Opin Neurobiol.* 27: 143–50.

Garey J., et al. (2002). Temporal and spatial quantitation of reproductive behaviors among mice housed in a seminatural environment. *Horm Behav.* 42: 294–306.
(2003). Genetic contributions to generalized arousal of brain and behavior. *Proc Natl Acad Sci U S A.* 100(19): 11019–22.

Gaus S. E., et al. (2002). Ventrolateral preoptic nucleus contains sleep-active, galaninergic neurons in multiple mammalian species. *Neuroscience.* 115(1): 285–94.

Gennarelli T. A, et al. (1982). Diffuse axonal injury and traumatic coma in the primate. *Ann Neurol.* 12: 564–74.

Gerashchenko D., Kohls M. D., Greco M., et al. (2001). Hypocretin-2-saporin lesions of the lateral hypothalamus produce narcoleptic-like sleep behavior in the rat. *J Neurosci.* 21: 7273–83.

Gezelius H., López-Bendito G. (2017). Thalamic neuronal specification and early circuit formation. *Dev Neurobiol.* 77(7): 830–43.

Giacino J., Fins J. J., Machado A., Schiff N. D. (2012). Central thalamic deep brain stimulation to promote recovery from chronic posttraumatic minimally conscious state: challenges and opportunities. *Neuromodulation.* 15(4): 339–49.

Giacino J. T., Kalmar K., Whyte J. (2004). The JFK Coma Recovery Scale-Revised: measurement characteristics and diagnostic utility. *Arch Phys Med Rehab.* 85: 2020–9.

Giacino J. T., et al. (2014). Disorders of consciousness after acquired brain injury: the state of the science. *Nature Rev Neurol.* 10(2): 99–114.

Gilbert K. A., Lydic R. (1990). Parabrachial neuron discharge in the cat is altered during the carbachol-induced REM sleep-like state (DCarb) *Neurosci Lett.* 120: 241–4.

Gillies G. E., McArthur S. (2010). Estrogen actions in the brain and the basis for differential action in men and women: a case for sex-specific medicines. *Pharmacological Rev.* 62(2): 155–98.

Gloor P., Ball G., Schaul N. (1977). Brain lesions that produce delta waves in the EEG. *Neurology.* 27(4): 326–33.

Gogos J., et al. (1998). Catechol-O-methyltransferase-deficient mice exhibit sexually dimorphic changes in catecholamine levels and behavior. *Proc Natl Acad Sci U S A.* 95: 9991–6.

Goldfoot D., Baum M. Initiation of mating behavior in developing male rats following peripheral electric shock. *Physiol Behav.* 8: 857–63.

González-Cuello A., Milanés M. V., Laorden M. L. (2004). Increase of tyrosine hydroxylase levels and activity during morphine withdrawal in the heart. *Eur J Pharmacol.* 506(2): 119–28.

Gooley J. J., Schomer A., Saper C. B. (2006). The dorsomedial hypothalamic nucleus is critical for the expression of food-entrainable circadian rhythms. *Nat Neurosci.* 9(3): 398–407.

Graham M. D., Pfaus J. G. (2012). The effect of specific dopamine receptor antagonists in the medial preoptic area on the sexual behaviour of female rats. *Pharmacol Biochem Behav.* 102: 532–9.

Greco M. A., Fuller P. M., Jhou T. C., et al. (2008). Opioidergic projections to sleep-active neurons in the ventrolateral preoptic nucleus. *Brain Res.* 1245: 96–107.

Gregg T. R. (2003). Cortical and limbic neural circuits mediating aggressive behavior. In: Mattson M. P. (Ed.), *Neurobiology of Aggression.* Totowa, NJ: Humana Press, pp. 1–21.

Gritti I., et al. (2006). Stereological estimates of the basal forebrain cell population in the rat, including neurons containing choline acetyltransferase, glutamic acid decarboxylase or phosphate-activated glutaminase and colocalizing vesicular glutamate transporters. *Neuroscience.* 143(4): 1051–64.

Groenewegen H. J., Berendse H. W. (1994). The specificity of the 'nonspecific' midline and intralaminar thalamic nuclei. *Trends Neurosci.* 17(2): 52–7.

Grove E. A. (1988). Neural associations of the substantia innominata in the rat: afferent connections. *J Comp Neurol.* 277: 315–46.

Guarraci F. A. (2010). Sex, drugs and the brain: the interaction between drugs of abuse and sexual behavior in the female rat. *Horm Behav.* 58(1): 138–48.

Guiard B. P., et al. (2008). Functional interactions between dopamine, serotonin and norepinephrine neurons. *Int J Neuropsychopharmacol.* 11: 625–39.

Gulia K. K., Mallick H. N., Kumar V. M. (2003). Orexin A (hypocretin-1) application at the medial preoptic area potentiates male sexual behavior in rats. *Neuroscience.* 116(4): 921–3.

Guyenet P., et al. (1996). Role of medulla oblongata in generation of sympathetic and vabal outflows. In: Holstege G., Bandler R., Saper C.B., (1996). The Emotional Motor System: Progress in Brain Research Vol. 107. Elsevier

Hadj-Bouziane F., et al. (2012). Amygdala lesions disrupt modulation of functional MRI activity evoked by facial expression in the monkey inferior temporal cortex. *Proc Natl Acad Sci U S A.* 109(52):E3640–8.

Hadjimarkou M. M., et al. (2008). Estradiol suppresses rapid eye movement sleep and activation of sleep-active neurons in the ventrolateral preoptic area. *Eur J Neurosci.* 27(7): 1780–92.

Hagemann D., Waldstein S. R., Thayer J. F. (2003). Central and autonomic nervous system integration in emotion. *Brain Cogn.* 52(1): 79–87.

Haglund L., Köhler C., Ross S. B., Kelder D. (1979). Forebrain projections of the ventral tegmentum as studied by axonal transport of [3H]dopamine in the rat. *Neurosci Lett.* 12: 301–6.

Hagmann P., et al. (2008). Mapping the structural core of human cerebral cortex. *PLoS Biol.* 6(7):e159.

Hall, J. C., Rosbash M. (1988). Mutations and molecules influencing biological rhythms. *Ann Rev Neurosci.* 11: 373–93.

Han W., et al. (2017a). Integrated control of predatory hunting by the central nucleus of the amygdala. *Cell.* 168(1–2):311–24.

Han X., et al. (2017b). Role of dopamine projections from ventral tegmental area to nucleus accumbens and medial prefrontal cortex in reinforcement behaviors assessed using optogenetic manipulation. *Metab Brain Dis.* doi: 10.1007/s11011-017-0023-3.

Hansen S., et al. (2017). Testosterone influences volitional, but not reflexive orienting of attention in human males. *Physiol Behav.* 175: 82–7.

Harris G. C., Aston-Jones G. (2006). Arousal and reward: a dichotomy in orexin function. *Trends Neurosci.* 29(10): 571–7.

Harris C. W., Edwards J. L., Baruch A., et al. (2000). Effects of mental stress on brachial artery flow-mediated vasodilation in healthy normal individuals. *Am Heart J.* 139:405–11.

Harrison L. A., Hurlemann R., Adolphs R. (2015). An enhanced default approach bias following amygdala lesions in humans. *Psychonomic Sci.* 26: 1543–55.

Hasenstaub A., Shu Y., Haider B., et al. (2005). Inhibitory postsynaptic potentials carry synchronized frequency information in active cortical networks. *Neuron.* 47: 423–35.

Haubensak W., et al. (2010). Genetic dissection of an amygdala microcircuit that gates conditioned fear. *Nature.* 468: 270–5.

He B. J. (2014). Scale-free brain activity: past, present, and future. *Trends Cogn Sci.* 18(9): 480–7.

(2008). Electrophysiological correlates of the brain's intrinsic large-scale functional architecture. *PNAS.* 105: 16039–44.

Hebb D. O. (1955). Drives and the CNS. *Psych Rev.* 62: 243–54.

Heesink L., et al. (2017). Anger and aggression problems in veterans are associated with an increased acoustic startle reflex. *Biol Psychol.* 123: 119–25.

Hemmings H. C., Hopkins P. M. (2006). *Foundations of Anesthesia* (2nd edition). Philadelphia, PA: Mosby/Elsevier.

Herbert H., Saper C. B. (1992). Organization of medullary adrenergic and noradrenergic projections to the periaqueductal gray matter in the rat. *J Comp Neurol.* 315(1): 34–52.

Hermann G. E., Rogers R. C. (1985). Convergence of vagal and gustatory afferent input within the parabrachial nucleus of the rat. *J Auton Nerv Syst.* 13(1): 1–17.

Herold K. F., Andersen O. S., Hemmings H. C., Jr. (2017). Divergent effects of anesthetics on lipid bilayer properties and sodium channel function. *Eur Biophys J.* doi: 10.1007/s00249-017-1239-1.

Hesse J., Gross T. (2014). Self-organized criticality as a fundamental property of neural systems. *Front Syst Neurosci.* 8: 1–14.

Heyne H. O., Lautenschläger S., Nelson R., et al. (2014) Genetic influences on brain gene expression in rats selected for tameness and aggression. *Genetics.* 198:1277–1290

Hill, C. (2009). *Consciousness.* Cambridge: University of Cambridge Press.

Hiroi R., Neumaier J. F. (2006). Differential effects of ovarian steroids on anxiety versus fear as measured by open field test and fear-potentiated startle. *Behav Brain Res.* 166(1): 93–100.

Hobson J. A., Scheibel A. B. (1980). The brainstem core: sensorimotor integration and behavioral state control. *Neurosci Res Program Bull.* 18(1): 1–173.

Hodgins M. B., Spike R. C., Mackie R. M., MacLean A. B. (1998). An immunohistochemical study of androgen, oestrogen and progesterone receptors in the vulva and vagina. *British J Obstet Gynaecol.* 105: 216–22.

Holder M. K., et al. (2010). Methamphetamine facilitates female sexual behavior and enhances neuronal activation in the medial amygdala and ventromedial nucleus of the hypothalamus. *Psychoneuroendocrinology.* 35(2): 197–208.

Holder M. K., Mong J. A. (2010). Methamphetamine enhances paced mating behaviors and neuroplasticity in the medial amygdala of female rats. *Horm Behav.* 58(3): 519–25.

Holder M. K., Veichweg S. S., Mong J. A. (2015). Methamphetamine-enhanced female sexual motivation is dependent on dopamine and progesterone signaling in the medial amygdala. *Horm Behav.* 67: 1–11.

Horney C. J., et al. (2009). Predicting human resting-state functional connectivity from structural connectivity. *PNAS.* 106: 2035–40.

Horvitz J. C. (2000). Mesolimbocortical and nigrostriatal dopamine responses to salient non-reward events. *Neuroscience.* 96(4): 651–6.

Hucho T. B., Dina O. A., Kuhn J., Levine J. D. (2006). Estrogen controls PKCepsilon-dependent mechanical hyperalgesia through direct action on nociceptive neurons. *Eur J Neurosci.* 24(2): 527–34.

Hudson A. E., Calderon D. P., Pfaff D. W., Proekt A. (2014). Recovery of consciousness is mediated by a network of discrete metastable activity states. *Proc Natl Acad Sci U S A.* 111(25): 9283–8.

Hull E. (2016). Male sexual behavior. In: Pfaff D., Joels M. (Eds.), *Hormones, Brain and Behavior.* Cambridge: Academic Press/Elsevier, pp. 1–45.

Hull E. M., Dominguez J. M. (2006). Getting his act together: roles of glutamate, nitric oxide, and dopamine in the medial preoptic area *Brain Res.* 1126(1): 66–75.

Humphrey N. (1992). *A History of the Mind.* New York, NY: Copernicus/Springer Verlag. (2011). *Soul Dust: The Magic of Consciousness.* Princeton, NJ: Princeton University Press.

Hungs M., et al. (2001). Identification and functional analysis of mutations in the hypocretin (orexin) genes of narcoleptic canines. *Genome Res.* 11: 531–9.

Hungs M., Lin L., Okun M., Mignot E. (2001). Polymorphisms in the vicinity of the hypocretin/orexin are not associated with human narcolepsy. *Neurology.* 57(10): 1893–5.

Iams S. G., Wexler B. C. (1979). Inhibition of the development of spontaneous hypertension in SH rats by gonadectomy or estradiol. *J Lab Clin Med.* 94(4): 608–16.

Ishizuka T., Murotani T., Yamatodani A. (2012). Action of modafinil through histaminergic and orexinergic neurons. *Vitamins Hormones.* 89: 259–78.

Ito K., Yanagihara M., Imon H., Dauphin L., McCarley R. W. (2002). Intracellular recordings of pontine medial gigantocellular tegmental field neurons in the naturally sleeping cat: behavioral state-related activity and soma size difference in order of recruitment. *Neuroscience.* 114(1): 23–37.

Jack A. I., et al. (2013). fMRI reveals reciprocal inhibition between social and physical cognitive domains. *Neuroimage.* 66: 385–401.

Jacobs B. L., Fornal C. A., (2010). Activity of brain serotonergic neurons in relation to physiology and behavior. In: Muller C., Jacobs B. (Eds.), *Handbook of Behavioral Neurobiology of Serotonin.* San Diego, CA: Elsevier/Academic Press, pp. 153–62.

James W. *The Principles of Psychology* (volume 2). New York, NY: Dover (1890, reprinted 1950).

Jankowski M., Rachelska G., Donghao W., et al. (2001). Estrogen receptors activate atrial natriuretic peptide in the rat heart. *Proc Natl Acad Sci U S A.* 98: 11765–70.

Jasper H. (Ed.). (1958). *Reticular Formation of the Brain.* Detroit, MI: Symposium of the Henry Ford Hospital.

Jeong H. H., et al. (2000). The large scale organization of metabolic networks. *Nature.* 407: 651–4.

Jing J., Gillette R., Weiss K. R. (2009). Evolving concepts of arousal: insights from simple model systems. *Rev Neurosci.* 20(5–6):405–27.

Joel D., Weiner I. (1994). The organization of the basal ganglia-thalamocortical circuits: open interconnected rather than closed segregated. *Neuroscience.* 63(2): 363–79.

Johnson L. R., Hou M., Prager E. M., Ledoux J. E. (2011). Regulation of the fear network by mediators of stress: norepinephrine alters the balance between cortical and subcortical afferent excitation of the lateral amygdala. *Front Behav Neurosci.* 23(5): 23. doi: 10.3389/fnbeh.2011.00023.

Jones B. E. (1987). Retrograde labeling of neurones in the brain stem following injections of [3H]choline into the forebrain of the rat. *Exp Brain Res.* 65(2): 437–48. (2003). Arousal systems. *Front Biosci.* 8:s438–51. (2005). From waking to sleeping: neuronal and chemical substrates. *Trends Pharmacol Sci.* 26(11): 578–86.

Jones B. E., Beaudet A. (1987) Article I. Retrograde labeling of neurones in the brain stem following injections of [3H]choline into the forebrain of the rat. *Exp Brain Res.* 65(2): 437–48.

Jones B. E., Cuello A. C. (1989). Afferents to the basal forebrain cholinergic cell area from pontomesencephalic – catecholamine, serotonin, and acetylcholine – neurons. *Neuroscience.* 31: 37–61.

Jones B. E., Yang T. Z. (1985). The efferent projections from the reticular formation and the locus coeruleus studied by anterograde and retrograde axonal transport in the rat. *J Comp Neurol.* 242: 56–92.

Kagan J., Snidman N. (1999). Early childhood predictors of adult anxiety disorders. *Biol Psychiatry.* 46(11): 1536–41.

Kahneman D. and Tversky, A. (2011). *Thinking Fast and Slow.* New York, NY: Farrar, Straus & Giroux.

Kaiser M. (2011). A tutorial in connectome analysis: topological and spatial features of brain networks. *Neuroimage.* 57(3): 892–907.

Kampfl A., et al. (1998). The persistent vegetative state after closed head injury: clinical and magnetic resonance imaging findings in 42 patients. *J Neurosurg.* 88: 809–16.

Kandel, E. (2000). *Principles of Neural Science* (4th edition). New York, NY: McGraw-Hill.

Kandel E. (2012). *The Age of Insight.* NewYork, NY: Random House.

Kapas L., Obal F., Jr, Book A. A., et al. (1996). The effects of immunolesions of nerve growth factor-receptive neurons by 192 IgG-saporin on sleep. *Brain Res.* 712: 53–9.

Karatsoreos I., Silver R. (2007). The neuroendocrinology of the suprachiasmatic nucleus as a conductor of body timer in mammals. *Endocrinology.* 148: 5640–7.

Karatsoreos I. N., et al. (2011). Androgens modulate structure and function of the suprachiasmatic nucleus brain clock. *Endocrinology.* 152(5): 1970–8.

Kaur S., Junek A., Black M. A., Semba K. (2008). Effects of ibotenate and 192IgG-saporin lesions of the nucleus basalis magnocellularis/substantia innominata on spontaneous sleep and wake states and on recovery sleep after sleep deprivation in rats. *J Neurosci.* 28(2): 491–504.

Kaur S., et al. (2013). Glutamatergic signaling from the parabrachial nucleus plays a critical role in hypercapnic arousal. *J Neurosci.* 33(18): 7627–40.

Keenan D. M., Quinkert A. W., Pfaff D. W. (2015). Stochastic modeling of mouse motor activity under deep brain stimulation: the extraction of arousal information. *PLoS Comput Biol.* 11(2):e1003883. doi: 10.1371/journal.pcbi.1003883.

Keizer K., Kuypers H. G. (1989). Distribution of corticospinal neurons with collaterals to lower brain stem reticular formation in cat. *Experimental Brain Res.* 54(1): 107–20.

Kennedy A., et al. (2014). Internal states and behavioral decision-making: toward an integration of emotion and cognition. *Cold Spring Harb Symp Quant Biol.* 79: 199–210.

Kidd P. B., Young M. W., Siggia E. D. (2015). Temperature compensation and temperature sensation in the circadian clock. *Proc Natl Acad Sci U S A.* 112(46):E6284–92.

Kim J. W., Closs E. I., Albritton L. M., Cunningham J. M. (1991). Transport of cationic amino acids by the mouse ecotropic retrovirus receptor. *Nature.* 352:725–8.

King G. W. (1980). Topology of ascending brainstem projections to nucleus parabrachialis in the cat. *J Comp Neurol.* 191(4): 615–38.

Kitamura T., et al. (2017). Engrams and circuits crucial for systems consolidation of a memory. *Science.* 356: 73–78.

Koch C. (2008). In: Squire L. R., et al. (Eds.), *Fundamental Neuroscience.* San Diego, CA: Academic Press (Elsevier), pp. 1223–35.

Koch K. (2017). How to make a consciousness meter. *Scientific American*, November, pp. 28–34.

Kojima T., et al. (2009). Default mode of brain activity demonstrated by positron emission tomography imaging in awake monkeys: higher rest-related than working memory-related activity in medial cortical areas. *J Neurosci.* 29(46): 14463–71.

Kolber Benedict J., et al. (2008). Central amygdala glucocorticoid receptor action promotes fear-associated CRH activation and conditioning. *Proc Natl Acad Sci U S A.* 105(33): 12004–9.

Konopka R. J., Benzer, S. (1971a). Clock mutants of Drosophila melanogaster. *Proc Natl Acad Sci U S A.* 68(9): 2112–6. (1971b). Clock mutants of Drosophila melanogaster. *Proc Natl Acad Sci.* 68: 2112–18.

Korn H., Faber, D. S. (2005). The Mauthner cell half a century later. *Neuron.* 47: 13–28.

Kow L.-M., Pfaff, D. W. (1973). Effects of estrogen treatment on the size of receptive field and response threshold of pudendal nerve in the female rat. *Neuroendocrinology,* 13:299–313.

Koyama M., et al. (2011). Mapping a sensory-motor network onto a structural and functional ground plan in the hindbrain. *Proc Natl Acad Sciences U S A.* 108(3): 1170–5.

Kreibich A., et al. (2008). Presynaptic inhibition of diverse afferents to the locus ceruleus by kappa-opiate receptors: a novel mechanism for regulating the central norepinephrine system. *J Neurosci.* 28(25): 6516–25.

Krout K. E., Loewy A. D. (2000). Parabrachial nucleus projections to midline and intralaminar thalamic nuclei of the rat. *J Comp Neurol.* 428: 475–94.

Kume K., Kume S., Park S. K., Hirsh J., Jackson F. R. (2005). Dopamine is a regulator of arousal in the fruit fly. *J Neurosci.* 25(32): 7377–84.

Kumral E., Evyapan D., Balkör K., Kutluhan S. (2001). Bilateral thalamic infarction. Clinical, etiological and MRI correlates. *Acta Neurol Scand.* 103: 35–42.

Kunkhyen T., et al. (2017). Optogenetic activation of accessory olfactory bulb input to the forebrain differentially modulates investigation of opposite versus same-sex urinary chemosignals and stimulates mating in male mice. *eNeuro.* 4(2) e0010–17.

Kuo H. J., Maslen C. L., Keene D. R., Glanville R. W. (1997). Type VI collagen anchors endothelial basement membranes by interacting with type IV collagen. *J Biol Chem.* 272:26522–9.

Kurata J., Hemmings H. C. (2015). Memory and awareness in anaesthesia; the 9th international conference. *Br J Anesthesiol.* 115: Editorial, S1.

LaCroix-Fralish M. L., Tawfik V. L., DeLeo J. A. (2005). The organizational and activational effects of sex hormones on tactile and thermal hypersensitivity following lumbar nerve root injury in male and female rats. *Pain.* 114(1–2):71–80.

LaLumiere R. T., McGaugh J. L., McIntyre C. K. (2017). Emotional modulation of learning and memory: pharmacological implications. *Pharmacological Rev.* 69(3): 236–55.

Langton C. G. (1990). Computation at the edge of chaos. *Phys D.* 42: 12–37.

Lanuza E., Moncho-Bogani J., Ledoux J. E. (2008). Unconditioned stimulus pathways to the amygdala: effects of lesions of the posterior intralaminar thalamus on foot-shock-induced c-Fos expression in the subdivisions of the lateral amygdala. *Neuroscience.* 155(3): 959–68.

Laufs H. (2012). Functional imaging of seizures and epilepsy: evolution from zones to networks. *Curr Opin Neurol.* 25: 194–200.

Laumann T. O., et al. (2017). On the stability of BOLD fMRI correlations. *Cerebr Cortex.* 27: 4719–32.

Laureys S. (2016a). Traumatic brain damage: Severe brain damage, coma and disorders of consciousness. In: Pfaff D. W., Volkow N. D. (Eds.), *Neuroscience in the 21st Century* (2nd edition, volume 5). New York, NY: Springer Verlag, pp. 3341–70.
(2016b). Traumatic Brain Damage: Severe brain damage, coma and disorders of consciousness. In: Pfaff D., Volkow N., (Eds.), *Neuroscience in the 21st Century* (2nd edition, volume 5). New York, NY: Springer, pp. 3341–75.

Laureys, S. (2016). In: Pfaff D., Volkow N. (Eds.), *Neuroscience in the 21st Century* (volume 5), pp. 3341–71.

Laureys Steven, Schiff. Nicholas D. (2012). Coma and consciousness: paradigms (re) framed by neuroimaging. *Neuroimage.* 61: 478–91.

Ledo A., Frade J., Barbosa R. M., Laranjinha, J. (2004). Nitric oxide in brain: diffusion, targets and concentration dynamics in hippocampal subregions. *Mol Aspects Med.* 25:75–89.

LeDoux J. E. (2000). Emotion circuits in the brain. *Ann Rev Physiol.* 23: 155–84.
(2014). Coming to terms with fear. *Proc Natl Acad Sci.* 111: 2871–8.

LeDoux J. E., Brown R. (2017). A higher-order theory of emotional consciousness. *PNAS.* 114: 2016–25.

Lee M. G., Manns I. D., Alonso A., Jones B. E. (2004). Sleep–wake related discharge properties of basal forebrain neurons recorded with micropipettes in head-fixed rats. *J Neurophysiol.* 92: 1182–9.

Lee M. G., Hassani O. K., Alonso A., Jones B. E. (2005). Cholinergic basal forebrain neurons burst with theta during waking and paradoxical sleep. *J Neurosci.* 25(17): 4365–9.

Lee H.S., Kim M.A., and Waterhouse B.D., (2005). Retrograde double-labeling study of common afferent projections to the dorsal raphe and the nuclear core of the locus coeruleus in the rat. *J Comp Neurol.* 481: 179–93.

Lee A. W., et al. (2008). Estradiol modulation of phenylephrine-induced excitatory responses in ventromedial hypothalamic neurons of female rats. *Proc Natl Acad Sci U S A.* 105(20): 7333–8.

Lee H., et al. (2014). Scalable control of mounting and attack by Esr11 neurons in the ventromedial hypothalamus. *Nature.* 509: 627–32.

Lenaz G., Fato R., Genova M. L., et al. (2006). Mitochondrial Complex I: structural and functional aspects. *Biochim Biophys Acta.* 1757:1406–20.

Leontovich T. A., Zhukova G. P. (1963). The specificity of the neuronal structure and topography of the reticular formation in the brain and spinal cord of carnivora. *J Comp Neurol.* 121: 347–79.

Leresche N., Lambert R. C. (2017). GABA receptors and T-type Ca2+ channels crosstalk in thalamic networks. *Neuropharmacology.* pii:S0028-3908(17)30276-9.

LeSauter J., et al. (2009). Stomach ghrelin-secreting cells as food-entrainable circadian clocks. *Proc Natl Acad Sci U S A.* 106(32): 13582–7.

Levenson R. W. (2003). Blood, sweat and fears: the autonomic architecture of emotion. *Ann N Y Acad Sci.* 1000: 348–66.

Li H., Satinoff E. (1996). Body temperature and sleep in intact and ovariectomized female rats. *Am J Physiol.* 271(6 Pt 2):R1753–8.

Li S. B., Giardino W. J., de Lecea L. (2017). Hypocretins and arousal. *Curr Top Behav Neurosci.* 33: 93–104.

Li S. B., Jones J. R., de Lecea L. (2016). Hypocretins, neural systems, physiology, and psychiatric disorders. *Curr Psychiatry Rep.* 18(1): 7–14. doi: 10.1007/s11920-015-0639-0

Li A., et al. (2017). The fundamental advantages of temporal networks. *Science.* 358: 1042–52.

Liao Y., Smyth G. K., Shi, W. (2014). featureCounts: an efficient general purpose program for assigning sequence reads to genomic features. *Bioinformatics.* 30:923–30.

Lin D., Boyle M. P., Dollar P., et al. (2011). Functional identification of an aggression locus in the mouse hypothalamus. *Nature.* 470(7333): 221–6.

Lin L., Faraco J., Li R., et al. (1999). The sleep disorder canine narcolepsy is caused by a mutation in the hypocretin (orexin) receptor 2 gene. *Cell.* 98(3): 365–76.

Lin J. S., Anaclet C., Sergeeva O. A., and Haas H. L. (2011). The waking brain: an update. *Cell Mol Life Sci.* 68(15): 2499–512.

Lindsley D. B., Bowden J., Magoun H. W. (1949). Effect upon the EEG of acute injury to the brain stem activating system. *Electroencephalogr Clin Neurophysiol.* 1: 475–86.

Liu X., et al. (2016). Development of electrophysiological properties of nucleus gigantocellularis neurons correlated with increased CNS arousal. *Dev Neurosci.* 38(4): 295–310.

Liu Z.-P., et al. (2017). Delta subunit containing GABA-A receptor disinhibits lateral amygdala and facilitates fear expression in mice. *Biol Psychiatry.* 81: 990–1002.

Liu Y. Y., Barabasi, A.-L. Network science. *Rev Mod Phys.* 88(3): 035006–64.

Llinas R. R., Steriade M. (2006). Bursting of thalamic neurons and states of vigilance. *J Neurophysiol.* 95: 3297–308.

Loh S. Y., Salleh N. (2017). Influence of testosterone on mean arterial pressure: a physiological study in male and female normotensive WKY and hypertensive SHR rats. *Physiol Int.* 104(1): 25–34.

Loughlin S. E., Fallon J. H. (1982). Mesostriatal projections from ventral tegmentum and dorsal raphe: cells project ipsilaterally or contralaterally but not bilaterally. *Neurosci Lett.* 32(1): 11–6.

Lövblad K. O., Bassetti C., Mathis J., Schroth G. (1997). MRI of paramedian thalamic stroke with sleep disturbance. *Neuroradiology.* 39(10): 693–8.

Love M. I., Huber W., Anders S. (2014). Moderated estimation of fold change and dispersion for RNA-seq data with DESeq2. *Genome Biol.* 15:550.

Lovick T. A. (1993). The periaqueductal gray-rostral medulla connection in the defence reaction: efferent pathways and descending control mechanisms. *Behav Brain Res.* 58: 19–25.

(2016). Central control of visceral pain and urinary tract function. *Autonomic Neurosci.* 200: 35–42.

Lu J., Greco M. A., Shiromani P., Saper C. B. (2000). Effect of lesions of the ventrolateral preoptic nucleus on NREM and REM sleep. *J Neurosci.* 20: 3830–42.

Lu J., Bjorkum A. A., Xu M., et al. (2002). Selective activation of the extended ventrolateral preoptic nucleus during rapid eye movement sleep. *J Neurosci.* 22: 4568–76.

Lu J., Jhou T. C., Saper C. B. (2006). Identification of wake-active dopaminergic neurons in the ventral periaqueductal gray matter. *J Neurosci.* 26(1): 193–202.

Lu J., Nelson L. E., Franks N., et al. (2008). Role of endogenous sleep-wake and analgesic systems in anesthesia. *J Comp Neurol.* 508: 648–62.

Lu J., Sherman D., Devor M., Saper C. B. (2006). A putative flip-flop switch for control of REM sleep. *Nature.* 441: 589–94.

Lu Z. M., Li X. F. (2016). Attack vulnerability of network controllability. *PLoS One.* 11(9):e0162289. doi: 10.1371/journal. pone.0162289.

Luigetti M., Di Lazzaro V., Broccolini A., et al. (2011). Bilateral thalamic stroke transiently reduces arousals and NREM sleep instability. *J Neurol Sci.* 300: 151–4.

Lund T. D., Rovis T., Chung W. C., Handa R. J. (2005). Novel actions of estrogen receptor-beta on anxiety-related behaviors. *Endocrinology.* 146(2): 797–807.

Lunga P., Herbert J. (2004). 17Beta-oestradiol modulates glucocorticoid, neural and behavioural adaptations to repeated restraint stress in female rats. *J Neuroendocrinol.* 16(9): 776–85.

Luo A. H., Aston-Jones G. (2009). Circuit projection from suprachiasmatic nucleus to ventral tegmental area: a novel circadian output pathway. *Eur J Neurosci.* 10: 1–13.

Lutkenhoff E. S., et al. (2015). Thalamic and extra-thalamic mechanisms of consciousness after severe brain injury. *Ann Neurol.* 78: 68–76.

Ma S., et al. (2017). Dual-transmitter systems regulating arousal, attention, learning and memory. *Neurosci Biobehav Rev.* pii:S0149-7634(17)30066-0. doi: 10.1016/j.neubiorev.2017.07.009.

MacLeod N. K., Mayer M. L. (1980). Electrophysiological analysis of pathways connecting the medial preoptic area with the mesencephalic central grey matter in rats. *J Physiol.* 298: 53–70.

Magnasco M. (2003). A wave traveling over a Hopf instability shapes the cochlear tuning curve. *Phys Rev Lett.* 84: 243–6.

Magnasco M. O., Piro O., Cecchi G. A. (2009). Self-tuned critical anti-Hebbian networks. *Phys Rev Lett.* 102(25): 258102.

Magoun H. W. (1958). *The Waking Brain* (2nd edition). Springfield, IL: Charles C Thomas.

Mann K., et al. (2016). Immunity around the clock. *Science.* 354: 999–1009.

Manford M., Andermann F. (1998). Complex visual hallucinations. Clinical and neurobiological insights. *Brain.* :1819–40.

Marcus E. Raichle. (2006). The brain's dark energy. *Science.* 314: 1249–50.

Marcus J. N., et al. (2001). Differential expression of orexin receptors 1 and 2 in the rat brain. *J Comp Neurol.* 435(1): 6–25.

Marcus J. N., Aschkenasi C. J., Lee C. E., et al. (2001). Differential expression of orexin receptors 1 and 2 in the rat brain. *J Comp Neurol.* 435 (1):6–25.

Marin M. F., et al. (2017). Skin conductance responses and neural activations during fear conditioning and extinction recall across anxiety disorders. *JAMA Psychiatry.* 74(6): 622–31.

Markowitsch H. J., Irle E. (1981). Widespread cortical projections of the ventral tegmental area and of other brain stem structures in the cat. *Exp Brain Res.* 41: 233–46.

Marshall W., Albantakis L., Tononi G. (2018) Article I. Black-boxing and cause-effect power. *PLoS Comput Biol.* 14(4):e1006114. doi: 10.1371/journal.pcbi.1006114. eCollection 2018 Apr.

Martin E. M., Pavlides C., Pfaff D. (2010). Multimodal sensory responses of nucleus reticularis gigantocellularis and the responses' relation to cortical and motor activation. *J Neurophysiol.* 103(5): 2326–38.

Martin E. M., Devidze N., Shelley D. N., et al. (2011). Molecular and neuroanatomical characterization of single neurons in the mouse medullary gigantocellular

reticular neurons. *J Comp Neurol.* 519(13): 2574–93.

Martin-Alguacil N., Schober J. M., Kow L. M., Pfaff D. (2006). Arousing properties of the vulvar epithelium. *J Urol.* 176(2): 456–62.

Martin-Alguacil N., et al. (2008a). Clitoral sexual arousal: neuronal tracing study from the clitoris through the spinal tracts. *J Urol.* 180(4): 1241–8.

(2008b). Oestrogen receptor expression and neuronal nitric oxide synthase in the clitoris and prepucial gland structures of mice. *BJU Int.* 102(11): 1719–23.

Martin-Alguacil N., Pfaff D. W., Kow L. M., Schober J. M. (2008c). Oestrogen receptors and their relation to neural receptive tissue of the labia minora. *BJU Int.* 101(11): 1401–6.

Martin-Alguacil N., Pfaff D. W., Shelley D. N., Schober J. M. (2008d). Clitoral sexual arousal: an immunocytochemical and innervation study of the clitoris. *BJU Int.* 101(11): 1407–13.

Mason P., Leung C. (1996). Physiological functions of ontomedullary raphe and medial reticular neurons. In: Holstege G., et al. (Eds.), *Progress in Brain Research* (volume 107), pp. 269–81.

Mattson M. P. (2003). *Neurobiology of Aggression.* Totowa, NJ: Humana Press.

Matuszewich L., Lorrain D. S., Hull E. M. (2000). Dopamine release in the medial preoptic area of female rats in response to hormonal manipulation and sexual activity. *Behav Neurosci.* 114(4): 772–82.

McBride R. L., Sutin J. (1976). Projections of the locus coeruleus and adjacent pontine tegmentum in the cat. *J Comp Neurol.* 165(3): 265–84.

McCann J., Miyamoto S., Boyle C., Rogers K. (2007). Healing of hymenal injuries in prepubertal and adolescent girls: a descriptive study. *Pediatrics.* 119(5):e1094–106.

McCarthy E. A., et al. (2017). A comparison of the effects of male pheromone priming and optogenetic inhibition of accessory olfactory bulb forebrain inputs on the sexual behavior of estrous female mice. *Horm Behav.* 89: 104–12.

McCulloch W. S., Pitts W. (1943). A logical calculus of the ideas immanent in nervous activity. *Bull Math Biophys.* 5:115–33.

McDuffie J. E., Coaxum S. D., Maleque M. A. (1999). 5-Hydroxytryptamine evokes endothelial nitric oxide synthase activation in bovine aortic endothelial cell cultures. *Proc Soc Exp Biol Med.* 221:386–90.

Melloni R. H., Ricci L. A. (2010). Adolescent exposure to anabolic/androgenic steroids and the neurobiology of offensive aggression. *Horm Behav.* 58: 177–91.

Mena-Segovia J., Bolam J. P. (2017). Rethinking the pedunculopontine nucleus: from cellular organization to function. *Neuron.* 94(1): 7–18.

Mendelsohn M. E., Karas R. H. (1999). The protective effects of estrogen on the cardiovascular system. *New Engl J Med.* 340: 1801–11.

Menétrey D., De Pommery J. (1991). Origins of spinal ascending pathways that reach central areas involved in visceroception and visceronociception in the rat. *Eur J Neurosci.* 3(3): 249–59.

Meston C. M., Moe I. V., Gorzalka B. B.(1996). Effects of sympathetic inhibition on receptive, proceptive, and rejection behaviors in the female rat. *Physiol Behav.* 59: 537–42.

Metzinger T. (2002). *Neural Correlates of Consciousness.* Cambridge, MA: MIT Press.

Miczek K. A., Faccidomo S., De Almeida R. M., et al. (2004) Article I. Escalated aggressive behavior: new pharmacotherapeutic approaches and opportunities. *Ann NY Acad Sci.* 1036: 336–55.

Miller R. D. (Ed.). (2005). *Miller's Anesthesia* (6th edition) Philadelphia, PA: Churchill Livingstone/Elsevier.

Minert A., Yatziv S.-L., Devor M. (2017). Location of the mesopontine neurons responsible for maintenance of anesthetic loss of consciousness. *J Neurosci.* 37(38): 9320–31.

Misonou H., Mohapatra D. P., Trimmer J. S. (2005). Kv2.1: a voltage-gated k+ channel critical to dynamic control of neuronal excitability. *Neurotoxicology.* 26:743–52.

Mitchell, C. L. Kaelber, W. W. (1967). Unilateral vs bilateral medial thalamic lesions and reactivity to noxious stimuli. *Arch Neurol.* 17(6): 653–60.

Mitra C., et al. (2017). Multiple-node basin stability in complex dynamical networks. *Phys Rev E.* 95(3–1):032317. doi: 10.1103.

Mlinar B., et al. (2016). Firing properties of genetically identified dorsal raphe serotonergic neurons in brain slices. *Front Cell Neurosci.* 10:195. Doi: 10.3389/fncel.2016.00195.

Model Z., et al. (2015). Suprachiasmatic nucleus as the site of androgen action on circadian rhythms. *Horm Behav.* 73: 1–7.

Moga M. M., Herbert H., Hurley K. M., et al. (1990). Organization of cortical, basal forebrain, and hypothalamic afferents to the parabrachial nucleus in the rat. *J Comp Neurol.* 295: 624–61.

Mong J. A., et al. (2003a). Estradiol differentially regulates lipocalin-type prostaglandin D synthase transcript levels in the rodent brain: evidence from high-density oligonucleotide arrays and in situ hybridization. *Proc Natl Acad Sci U S A.* 100(1): 318–23.

Mong J. A., Devidze N., Goodwillie A., Pfaff D. W. (2003b). Reduction of lipocalin-type prostaglandin D synthase in the preoptic area of female mice mimics estradiol effects on arousal and sex behavior. *Proc Natl Acad Sci U S A.* 100(25): 15206–11.

Mong J. A., et al. (2011). Sleep, rhythms, and the endocrine brain: influence of sex and gonadal hormones. *J Neurosci.* 31(45): 16107–16.

Monti M. M., et al. (2015). Thalamo-frontal connectivity mediates top-down cognitive functions in disorders of consciousness. *Neurology.* 84: 167–73.

Monti Martin M. (2016). Non-invasive ultrasonic thalamic stimulation in disorders of consciousness after severe brain injury: a first-in-man report. *Brain Stimul.* 9: 940–1.

Moore R. Y., Abrahamson E. A., Van Den Pol A. (2001). The hypocretin neuron system: an arousal system in the human brain. *Arch Ital Biol.* 139(3): 195–205.

Morgan M., Pfaff D. (2001) Effects of estrogen on activity and fear-related behaviors in mice. *Horm. Behav.* 40:472–482

Morin L.P. (2013) Neuroanatomy of the extended circadian rhythm system. *Exp Neurol.* 243: 4–20. doi: 10.1016/j.expneurol.2012.06.026. Epub 2012 Jul 2.

Morison R. S., Dempsey E. W. (1942). A study of thalamo-cortical relations. *Am J Physiol.* 135: 281–92.

Morrell J. I., Pfaff D. W. (1983). Retrograde hrp identification of neurons in the rhombencephalon and spinal cord of the rat that project to the dorsal mesencephalon. *Am J Anat.* 167: 229–40.

Morrell J. I., Greenberger L. M., Pfaff D. W. (1981). Hypothalamic, other diencephalic, and telencephalic neurons that project to the dorsal midbrain. *J Comp Neurol.* 201: 589–620.

Moruzzi G., Magoun H. (1949). Brain stem reticular formation and activation of the EEG. *Electroencephalogr Clin Neurophysiol.* 1: 455–73. [PubMed]

Motta S. C., et al. (2017). The periaqueductal gray and primal emotional processing critical to influence complex defensive responses, fear learning and reward seeking. *Neurosci Biobehav Rev.* 76(Pt A):39–47.

Motter A. E. (2004). Cascade control and defense in complex networks. *Phys Rev Lett.* 93(9): 098701.

Mountcastle V. B. (1974). *Mountcastle, VB Medical Physiology* (13th edition). St Louis, MO: Mosby, pp. 254–84.

Mukouyama Y. S., Gerber H. P., Ferrara N., Gu C., Anderson D. J. (2005). Peripheral nerve-derived VEGF promotes arterial differentiation via neuropilin 1-mediated positive feedback. *Development.* 132(5): 941–52.

Munk M. H., Roelfsema P. R., Konig P., Engel A. K., Singer W. (1996). Role of reticular activation in the modulation of intracortical synchronization. *Science.* 272: 271–4.

Muoio V., Persson P. B., Sendeski M. M. (2014). The neurovascular unit – concept review. *Acta Physiol (Oxf).* 210:790–8.

Murphy C. P., et al. (2017). MicroRNA-mediated rescue of fear extinction memory by miR 144-3p in extinction-impaired mice. *Biol Psychiatry.* 81: 979–89.

Muschamp J. W., et al. (2007). A role for hypocretin (orexin) in male sexual behavior. *J Neuroscience.* 27(11): 2837–45.

Myers B., et al. (2017). Ascending mechanisms of stress integration: implications for brainstem regulation of neuroendocrine and behavioral stress responses. *Neurosci Biobehav Rev.* 74(Pt B):366–75.

Nakajima M., Halassa M. M. (2017). Thalamic control of functional cortical connectivity. *Curr Opin Neurobiol.* 44: 127–31.

Nauta W. J. H. (1946). Hypothalamic regulation of sleep in rats. Experimental study. *J Neurophysiol.* 9: 285–316.

Nauta W. J. H., Kuypers H. G. J. M. (1958). Some ascending pathways in the brainstem reticular formation. In: Jasper H. (Ed.), *The Reticular Formation of the Brain.* Boston, MA: Little Brown, pp. 3–30.

Nautiyal K. M., Hen R. (2017). Serotonin receptors in depression: from A to B. *F1000Res.* 6:123. doi: 10.12688/f1000research.9736.1.

Nectow A. R., Ekstrand M. I., Friedman J. M. (2015). Molecular characterization of neuronal cell types based on patterns of projection with Retro-TRAP. *Nat Protoc.* 10:1319–27.

Nelson R. (Ed.). (2006). *Biology of Aggression.* Oxford: Oxford University Press.

Ng R. C., et al. (2010). Pharmacologic treatment for postpartum depression: a systematic review. *Pharmacotherapy.* 30(9): 928–41.

Nickenig G., Strehlow K., Wassmann S., et al. (2000). Differential effects of estrogen and progesterone on AT(1) receptor gene expression in vascular smooth muscle cells. *Circulation.* 102: 1828–33.

Nicoll R. A. (2017). A brief history of long-term potentiation. *Neuron.* 93:281–90.

Nishino S., et al. (2000). Hypocretin (orexin) transmission is defective in human narcolepsy. *Lancet.* 355: 39–40. (2001). Low cerebrospinal fluid hypocretin (Orexin) and altered energy homeostasis in human narcolepsy. *Ann Neurol.* 50(3): 381–8.

Nomura M., Durback L., Chan J., et al. (2002). Genotype/age interactions on aggressive behavior in gonadally intact estrogen receptor β knockout (βERKO) male mice. *Horm Behav.* 41(3): 288–96.

Norton L., et al. (2012). Disruptions of functional connectivity in the default mode network of comatose patients. *Neurology.* 78: 175–81.

Nyberga L., et al. (2010). Consciousness of subjective time in the brain. *PNAS.* 107: 22356–9.

Ogawa S., et al. (1998a). Roles of estrogen receptor-alpha gene expression in reproduction-related behaviors in female mice. *Endocrinology.* 139(12): 5070–81. (1998b). Modifications of testosterone-dependent behaviors by estrogen receptor-alpha gene disruption in male mice. *Endocrinology.* 139: 5058–69.

Ogawa S., Chan J., Gustafsson J. A., Korach K. S., Pfaff D. W. (2003). Estrogen increases locomotor activity in mice through estrogen receptor alpha: specificity for the type of activity. *Endocrinology.* 144(1): 230–9.

Ogawa S., Choleris E., Pfaff D. (2004). Genetic influences on aggressive behaviors and arousability in animals. *Ann N Y Acad Sci.* 1036: 257–66.

Ogawa S., Nomura M., Choleris E., Pfaff D., in Nelson (op cit., 2006). The roles of estrogen receptors in the regulation of aggressive behaviors. pp.231–250

Oloyo A. K., et al. (2016). Orchidectomy attenuates high-salt diet-induced increases in blood pressure, renovascular resistance, and hind limb vascular dysfunction: role of testosterone. *Clin Exp Pharmacol Physiol.* 43(9): 825–33.

Ott E., et al. (1994). *Coping with Chaos: Analysis of Chaotic Data and the Exploitation of Chaotic Systems.* New York, NY: Wiley.

Owen A. M., Coleman M. R. (2008a). Functional neuroimaging of the vegetative state. *Nat Rev Neurosci.* 9(3): 235–43. (2008b). Using neuroimaging to detect awareness in disorders of consciousness. *Funct Neurol.* 23(4): 189–94.

Owen A. M., et al. (2006). Detecting awareness in the vegetative state. *Science.* 313(5792): 1402.

Pace-Schott E. F., et al. (2008). In: Squire L. R., et al. (Eds.), *Fundamental Neuroscience.* San Diego, CA: Academic Press (Elsevier), pp. 958–85.

Palmer R. M., Ashton D. S., Moncada S. (1988). Vascular endothelial cells synthesize nitric oxide from L-arginine. *Nature.* 333:664–6.

Panksepp J. (1998). *Affective Neuroscience.* New York, NY: Oxford University Press.

Panula P., et al. (2015). International union of basic and clinical pharmacology. XCVIII. Histamine receptors. *Pharmacol Rev.* 67(3): 601–55.

Papka R. E., Srinivasan B., Miller K. E., Hayashi S. (1997). Localization of estrogen receptor protein and estrogen receptor messenger RNA in peripheral autonomic and sensory neurons. *Neuroscience.* 79: 1153–63.

Park K. K., Liu K., Hu Y., et al. (2008). Promoting axon regeneration in the adult CNS by modulation of the PTEN/mTOR pathway. *Science.* 322:963–6.

Parvizi J., Damasio A. R. (2003). Neuroanatomical correlates of brainstem coma. *Brain.* 126: 1524–36.

Paulauskis J. D., Sul H. S. (1989). Structure of mouse fatty acid synthase mRNA. Identification of the two NADPH binding sites. *Biochem Biophys Res Commun.* 158:690–5.

Paul M. J., Indic P., Schwartz W. J. (2011) Article I. A role for the habenula in the regulation of locomotor activity cycles. *Eur J Neurosci.* 34(3): 478-88. doi: 10.1111/j.1460-9568.2011.07762.x. Epub 2011 Jul 21.

Pauls S. D., et al. (2016). Deconstructing circadian rhythmicity with models and manipulations. *Trends Neurosci.* 39(6): 405–19.

Pereira de Vasconcelos A., Cassel J. C. (2015). The nonspecific thalamus: a place in a wedding bed for making memories last? *Neurosci Biobehav Rev.* 54: 175–96.

Perkins E., May P. J., Warren S. (2014). Feed-forward and feedback projections of midbrain reticular formation neurons in the cat. *Front Neuroanat.* 7: 55–71.

Peschanski M., Besson J. M. (1984). A spino-reticulo-thalamic pathway in the rat: an anatomical study with reference to pain transmission. *Neuroscience.* 12(1): 165–78.

Pessoa L., Ungerleider L. G. (2004). Neuroimaging studies of attention and the processing of emotion-laden stimuli. *Prog Brain Res.* 144: 171–82.

Peter Kuppens P., et al. (2016). The relation between valence and arousal in subjective experience varies with personality and culture. *J Pers.* 10: 1111–25.

Peterfi L., et al. (2004). Fos-immunoreactivity in the hypothalamus: dependency on the diurnal rhythm, sleep, gender, and estrogen. *Neuroscience.* 124: 695–707.

Peterson B. W. (1979) Reticulospinal projections to spinal motor nuclei. *Annu Rev Physiol.* 41: 127–40.

Peterson B. W., Pitts N. G., Fukushima K. (1979). Reticulospinal connections with limb and axial motoneurons. *Exp Brain Res.* 36(1): 1–20.

Peyron C., et al. (2000). A mutation in early onset narcolepsy and a generalized absence of hypocretin peptides in human narcoleptic brains. *Nat Med.* 6: 991–7.

Pfaff D. (1999). *Drive*. Cambridge, MA: MIT Press.

(2006). *Brain Arousal and Information Theory*. Cambridge, MA: Harvard University Press.

(2014). *Altruistic Brain Theory*. New York, NY: Oxford University Press.

Pfaff D., Young L. (2014). *Frontiers in Neuroendocrinology: Sex Differences in Neurological and Psychiatric Disorders*. Amsterdam: Elsevier.

Pfaff D. W. (2006). *Brain Arousal and Information Theory: Neural and Genetic Mechanisms* (Cambridge, MA: Harvard University Press).

(2017). *How the Vertebrate Brain Regulates Behavior*. Cambridge, MA: Harvard University Press.

Pfaff D. W., Banavar J. R. (2007). A theoretical framework for CNS arousal. *BioEssays.* 29(8): 803–10.

Pfaff. D. W., Kieffer B. L. (Eds). (2008). Molecular and biophysical mechanisms of arousal, alertness and attention. *Ann N Y Acad Sci.* 1129: 1–15.

Pfaff D. W., Baum M. (2017). Hormone-dependent medial preoptic/lumbar spinal cord/autonomic coordination supporting male sexual behaviors. *Mol Cell Endocrinol.* 467:21–30. doi: 10.1016/j.mce.2017.10.018.

Pfaff D. W., et al. (2004). *Principles of Hormone/Behavior Relations* (2nd edition, 2018). San Diego, CA: Academic Press/Elsevier.

Pfaff D. W., Westberg L., Kow L. M. (2005). Generalized arousal of mammalian central nervous systems. *J Comp Neurol.* 493(1): 86–91.

Pfaff D. W., Kieffer B. L., Swanson L. W. (2008). Mechanisms for the regulation of state changes in the CNS. An introduction. *Ann N Y Acad Sci.* 1129:1–7.

Pfaff D. W., Rapin I., Goldman S. (2011). Male predominance in autism: neuroendocrine influences on arousal and social anxiety. *Autism Res.* 4(3): 163–76.

Pfaff D. W., Martin, E. M., Faber D. (2012). Origins of arousal: roles for medullary reticular neurons. *Trends Neurosci.* 35(8): 468–76.

Pfaff D. W., Gagnidze K., Hunter R. G. (2017). Molecular endocrinology of female reproductive behavior. *Mol Cell Endocrinol.* 467: 14–20. doi: 10.1016/j.mce.2017.10.019.

Pfaus J. G. (2010). Inhibitory and disinhibitory effects of psychomotor stimulants and depressants on the sexual behavior of male and female rats. *Horm Behav.* 58(1): 163–76.

Pfaus J. G., Pfaff D. W. (1992). Mu, delta, and kappa opioid receptor agonists selectively modulate sexual behaviors in the female rat: differential dependence on progesterone. *Horm Behav.* 26: 457–73.

Posner J., Russell J. A., Peterson B. S. (2005). The circumplex model of affect: an integrative approach to affective neuroscience, cognitive development, and psychopathology. *Dev Psychopathol.* 17(3): 715–34.

Posner J. B., Saper C. B., Schiff N. D., Plum F. (2007). *Diagnosis of Stupor and Coma* (volume 4). New York, NY: Oxford University Press, pp. 29–34.

Postfai M., Barabasi A.-L. (2017). Properties of scale-free networks. *Phys Rev E.* 94(3): 032316.

Presta A., Liu J., Sessa W. C., Stuehr D. J. (1997). Substrate binding and calmodulin binding to endothelial nitric oxide synthase coregulate its enzymatic activity. *Nitric Oxide.* 1:74–87.

Proekt A., Banavar J. R., Maritan A., Pfaff D. W. (2012). Scale invariance in the dynamics of spontaneous behavior. *Proc Natl Acad Sci.* 109(26): 10564–9.

Prouty E. W., Waterhouse B. D., Chandler D. J. (2017). Corticotropin releasing factor dose-dependently modulates excitatory synaptic transmission in the noradrenergic nucleus locus coeruleus. *Eur J Neurosci.* 45(5): 712–22.

Puzzo D., Staniszewski A., Deng S. X., et al. (2009). Phosphodiesterase 5 inhibition improves synaptic function, memory, and amyloid-beta load in an Alzheimer's disease mouse model. *J Neurosci.* 29:8075–86.

Quinkert A. W., Pfaff D. W. (2012). Temporal patterns of deep brain stimulation generated with a true random number generator and the logistic equation: effects on CNS arousal in mice. *Behav Brain Res.* 229(2): 349–58.

Quinkert A. W., Schiff N. D., Pfaff D. W. (2010). Temporal patterning of pulses during deep brain stimulation affects central nervous system arousal. *Behav Brain Res.* 214(2): 377–85.

Quinkert A. W., Vimal V., Reeke G., et al. (2011). Quantitative descriptions of generalized arousal, an elementary function of the vertebrate brain. *Proc Natl Acad Sci.* 108(Suppl. 3):15617–23.

Quirk G. J. (2016). Fear. In: Pfaff D. W., Volkow N. C. (Eds.), *Neuroscience in the 21st Century* (2nd edition). New York, NY: Springer, pp. 2412–35.

Rahman N., et al. (2018). Mathematical description of the phase transition from low to high behavioral activity. *Nature* (submitted).

Raichle M. E. (2010). Two views of brain function. *Trends Cogn Sci.* 14: 180–90. (2001). A default mode of brain function. *Proc Natl Acad Sci U S A.* 98(2): 676–82.

Raimondo F., et al. (2017). Brain–heart interactions reveal consciousness in noncommunicating patients. *Ann Neurol.* 82(4): 578–91.

Ramon-Moliner E., Nauta W. J. (1966). The isodendritic core of the brain stem. *J Comp Neurol.* 126:311–35.

Ranson S. W. (1939). Somnolence caused by hypothalamic lesions in monkeys. *Arch Neurol Psychiatr.* 41: 1–23.

Rasmussen J. J., et al. (2017). Increased blood pressure and aortic stiffness among abusers of anabolic androgenic steroids: potential effect of suppressed natriuretic peptides in plasma? *J Hypertension.* doi: 10.1097/HJH.0000000000001546.

Ravasz E., Barabási A. L. (2003). Hierarchical organization in complex networks. *Phys Rev E Stat Nonlin Soft Matter Phys.* 67(2 Pt 2):026112.

Ray S., Maunsell J. H. (2015). Do gamma oscillations play a role in cerebral cortex? *Trends Cogn Sci.* 19(2): 78–85.

Reddy P., et al. (1984). Molecular analysis of the period locus in *Drosophila melanogaster* and identification of a transcript involved in biological rhythms. *Cell.* 38(3): 701–10.

Reich P. B., Tjoelker M. G., Machado J-L., and Oleksyn J. (2006). Universal scaling of respiration, metabolism, size and nitrogen in plants. *Nature.* 439: 457–61.

Reyes B. A., Valentino R. J., Xu G., Van Bockstaele E. J. (2005). Hypothalamic projections to locus coeruleus neurons in rat brain. *Eur J Neurosci.* 22(1): 93–106.

Rhodes C. H., Morrell J. I., Pfaff D. W. (1982). Estrogen-concentrating neurophysin-containing hypothalamic magnocellular neurons in the vasopressin-deficient (Brattleboro) rat: a study combining steroid autoradiography and immunocytochemistry. *J Neurosci.* 2: 1718–24.

Ribeiro A. C., et al. (2007). Two forces for arousal: Pitting hunger versus circadian influences and identifying neurons responsible for changes in behavioral arousal. *Proc Natl Acad Sci U S A.* 104(50): 20078–83.

Ribeiro A. C., Pfaff D. W., Devidze N. (2009). Estradiol modulates behavioral arousal and induces changes in gene expression profiles in brain regions involved in the control of vigilance. *Eur J Neurosci.* 29(4): 795–801.

Rohaut B., Naccache L. (2017). Disentangling conscious from unconscious cognitive processing with event-related EEG potentials. *Rev Neurologie (Paris).* 173(7–8):521–8.

Romanov R. A., et al. (2017). Molecular interrogation of hypothalamic organization reveals distinct dopamine neuronal subtypes. *Nat Neurosci.* 20(2): 176–88.

Roozendaal B., et al. (1999). Basolateral amygdala noradrenergic influence enables enhancement of memory consolidation induced by hippocampal glucocorticoid receptor activation. *Proc Natl Acad Sci U S A.* 96(20): 11642–7.

Rowe D. C., Plomin R. (1977). Temperament in early childhood. *J Pers Assess.* 41(2): 150–6.

Russell J. A. (1980). A circumplex model of affect. *J Pers Social Psychol.* 39: 1151–78.

Saez L., Young M. W. (1988). In situ localization of the per clock protein during development of *Drosophila melanogaster. Mol Cell Biol.* 8(12): 5378–85.

Sakai K., et al. (1976). Afferent projections to the locus coeruleus nucleus in the cat. Study by the horseradish peroxidase technic. *C R Seances Soc Biol Fil.* 170(1): 115–19.

Sakurai T., et al. (1998). Orexin and orexin receptors: a family of hypothalamic neuropeptides and G-protein coupled receptors that regulate feeding behavior. *Cell.* 92: 573–85.

Sand R. M., et al. (2017). Isoflurane modulates activation and inactivation gating of the prokaryotic Na+ channel NaChBac. *J Gen Physiol.* 149(6): 623–38.

Saper C., et al. (2010). Sleep state switching. *Neuron.* 68: 1023–42.

Saper C. B. (1982). Reciprocal parabrachial-cortical connections in the rat. *Brain Res.* 242(1): 33–40. [PubMed]
(1984). Organization of cerebral cortical afferent systems in the rat. II. Magnocellular basal nucleus. *J Comp Neurol.* 222: 313–42.
(1985). Organization of cerebral cortical afferent systems in the rat. II. Hypothalamocortical projections. *J Comp Neurol.* 237: 21–46.
(2000). Brainstem modulation of sensation, movement and consciousness. In: Kandel E. R., et al. (Eds.), *Principles of Neural Science* (4th edition). New York, NY: McGraw-Hill, pp. 889–910.

Saper C. B., Loewy A. D. (1980). Efferent connections of the parabrachial nucleus in the rat. *Brain Res.* 197: 291–317.
(2016). Commentary on: efferent connections of the parabrachial nucleus in the rat. *Brain Res.* 1645: 15–17.

Saper C. B., Chou T. C., Scammell T. E. (2001). The sleep switch: hypothalamic control of sleep and wakefulness. *Trends Neurosci.* 24(12): 726–31.

Saper C. B., Scammell T. E., Lu J. (2005a). Hypothalamic regulation of sleep and circadian rhythms. *Nature.* 437: 1257–63.
(2005b). Hypothalamic regulation of sleep and circadian rhythms. *Nature.* 437: 1257–61.

Saper C. B., Fuller P. M., Pedersen N. P., Lu J., Scammell T. E. (2010). Sleep state switching. *Neuron.* 68(6): 1023–42.

Saper C. B., Loewy A. D., Swanson L. W., Cowan W. M. (1976) Article I. Direct hypothalamo-autonomic connections. *Brain Res.* 117(2): 305–12.

Sara S. J., Bouret S. (2012). Orienting and reorienting: the locus coeruleus mediates cognition through arousal. *Neuron.* 76: 130–41.

Sato, T. N., Tozawa, Y., Deutsch, U., et al. (1995). Distinct roles of the receptor tyrosine kinases Tie-1 and Tie-2 in blood vessel formation. *Nature.* 376: 70–4.

Scammell T. E., et al. (2000). Hypothalamic arousal regions are activated during modafinil-induced wakefulness. *J Neurosci.* 20(22): 8620–8.

Schaafsma S., Pfaff D. (2014). Etiologies underlying sex differences in Autism Spectrum Disorders. *Front Neuroendocrinol.* 35: 255–72.

Scheibel M., Scheibel A. (1961). Structural substrates for integrative patterns in the brain stem reticular core. In: Jasper H. (Ed.), *Reticular Formation of the Brain.* Boston, MA: Little, Brown, pp. 31–68.
(1961). On circuit patterns of the brain stem reticular core. *Annals N Y Acad Sci.* 89: 857–65.

Schiff N. D. (2005). Modeling the minimally conscious state: measurements of brain function and therapeutic possibilities. *Prog Brain Res.* 150: 473–93.
(2008). Central thalamic contributions to arousal regulation and neurological disorders of consciousness. *Ann N Y Acad Sci.* 1129: 105–18.
(2009). Recovery of consciousness after brain injury: a mesocircuit hypothesis. *Trends Neurosci.* 33: 1–9.
(2010). Recovery of consciousness after brain injury: a mesocircuit hypothesis. *Trends Neurosci.* 33(1): 1–9.
(2016). Central thalamic deep brain stimulation to support anterior forebrain mesocircuit function in the severely injured brain. *J Neural Transmission (Vienna).* 123(7): 797–806.

Schiff N. D., Plum F. (2000). The role of arousal and "gating" systems in the neurology of impaired consciousness. *J Clin Neurophysiol.* 17(5): 438–52.

Schiff N. D., et al. (2005). fMRI reveals large-scale network activation in minimally conscious patients. *Neurology.* 64: 514–23.
(2007). Behavioural improvements with thalamic stimulation after severe traumatic brain injury. *Nature.* 448: 600–5.

(2013). Gating of attentional effort through the central thalamus. *J Neurophysiol.* 109(4): 1152–63.

Schlosbeg H. (1954). Three dimensions of emotion. *Psychol Rev.* 61: 81–8.

Schmahmann J. D. (2003). Vascular syndromes of the thalamus. *Stroke.* 34(9): 2264–78.

Schmitt I., et al. (2017). Thalamic amplification of cortical connectivity sustains attentional control. *Nature.* 545: 219–23.

Schober J. M., Pfaff D. (2007). The neurophysiology of sexual arousal. *Best Pract Res Clin Endocrinol Metab.* 21(3): 445–61.

Schober J., Weil Z., Pfaff D. (2011). How generalized CNS arousal strengthens sexual arousal (and vice versa). *Horm Behav.* 59: 689–96.

Schölvinck M. L., et al. (2010). Neural basis of global resting-state fMRI activity. *Proc Natl Acad Sci U S A.* 107(22): 10238–43.

Schultz K. N., von Esenwein S. A., Hu M., et al. (2009) Article I. Viral vector-mediated overexpression of estrogen receptor-alpha in striatum enhances the estradiol-induced motor activity in female rats and estradiol-modulated GABA release. *J Neurosci.* 29(6): 1897–903. doi: 10.1523/JNEUROSCI.4647-08.2009.

Schultz W. (2015). Neuronal reward and decision signals: from theories to data. *Physiol Rev.* 95(3): 853–951.
(2016a). Dopamine reward prediction error coding. *Dialogues Clin Neurosci.* 18(1): 23–32.
(2016b). Dopamine reward prediction-error signalling: a two-component response. *Nat Rev Neurosci.* 17(3): 183–95.

Schwabe L., et al. (2013). Opposite effects of noradrenergic arousal on amygdala processing of fearful faces in men and women. *Neuroimage.* 73: 1–7.

Schwartz J. C. (2011). The histamine H3 receptor: from discovery to clinical trials with pitolisant. *Br J Pharmacol.* 163(4): 713–21.

Scott J. P. and Fuller J. L. (1965). *Genetics and the Social Behavior of the Dog.* Chicago, IL: University of Chicago Press.

Segarra A. C., et al. (2010). Estradiol: a key biological substrate mediating the response to cocaine in female rats. *Horm Behav.* 58(1): 33–43.

Sehgal A., Mignot E. (2011). Genetics of sleep and sleep disorders. *Cell.* 146: 194–207.

Senger D. R., Claffey K. P., Benes J. E., et al. (1997). Angiogenesis promoted by vascular endothelial growth factor: regulation through alpha1beta1 and alpha2beta1 integrins. *Proc Natl Acad Sci U S A.* 94:13612–17.

Senger D. R., Perruzzi C. A., Streit M., et al. (2002). The alpha(1)beta(1) and alpha(2) beta(1) integrins provide critical support for vascular endothelial growth factor signaling, endothelial cell migration, and tumor angiogenesis. *Am J Pathol.* 160:195–204.

Serova L., Rivkin M., Nakashima A., Sabban E. L. (2002). Estradiol stimulates gene expression of norepinephrine biosynthetic enzymes in rat locus coeruleus. *Neuroendocrinology.* 75(3): 193–200.

Serova L. I., Maharjan S., Sabban E. L. (2005). Estrogen modifies stress response of catecholamine biosynthetic enzyme genes and cardiovascular system in ovariectomized female rats. *Neuroscience.* 132(2): 249–59.

Shang Y., Griffith L. C., Rosbash M. (2008). Light-arousal and circadian photoreception circuits intersect at the large PDF cells of the *Drosophila* brain. *Proc Natl Acad Sci U S A.* 105(50): 19587–94.

Shannon C. (1948). A mathematical theory of communication. *Bell System Technical Journal.* 27: 379–397.

Sherin J. E., Elmquist J. K., Torrealba F., Saper C. B. (1998). Innervation of histaminergic tuberomammillary neurons by GABAergic and galaninergic neurons in the ventrolateral preoptic nucleus of the rat. *J Neurosci.* 18: 4705–21.

Sherin J. E., Shiromani P. J., McCarley R. W., Saper C. B. (1996). Activation of ventrolateral preoptic neurons during sleep. *Science.* 271(5246): 216–9.

Shigemori M., et al. (1992). Coexisting diffuse axonal injury (DAI) and outcome of severe head injury. *Acta Neurochir Suppl (Wien).* 55: 37–9.

Shirvalkar P., et al. (2006). Cognitive enhancement with central thalamic electrical stimulation. *PNAS.* 103: 17007–12.

Shouse M. N., Siegel J. M. (1992). Pontine regulation of REM sleep components in cats: integrity of the pedunculopontine tegmentum (PPT) is important for phasic events but unnecessary for atonia during REM sleep. *Brain Res.* 571(1): 50–63.

Shulman G. L. et al. (1997). Common blood flow changes across visual tasks: decreases in cerebral cortex. *J Cogn Neurosci.* 95: 648–63.

Shulman R. G., Hyder F., Rothman D. L. (2009). Baseline brain energy supports the state of consciousness. *Proc Natl Acad Sci U S A.* 106(27): 11096–101.

Sieck G. C., Harper R. M. (1980). Discharge of neurons in the parabrachial pons related to the cardiac cycle: changes during different sleep-waking states. *Brain Res.* 199: 385–99.

Siegel J. (2004). Brain mechanisms that control sleep and waking. *Naturwissenschaften.* 8: 355–65.

Silver R., LeSauter J., Tresco P. A., Lehman M. N. (1996) Article II. A diffusible coupling signal from the transplanted suprachiasmatic nucleus controlling circadian locomotor rhythms. *Nature.* 382(6594): 810–3.

Simon H., Le Moal M., Calas, A. (1979). Efferents and afferents of the ventral tegmental-Al0 region studied after local injection of [3H] leucine and horseradish peroxidase. *Brain Res.* 178: 17–40.

Sinton C. M., McCarley R. W. (2004). Neurophysiological mechanisms of sleep and wakefulness: a question of balance. *Semin Neurol.* 24: 211–23.

Smith H. R., Pang K. C. (2005). Orexin-saporin lesions of the medial septum impair spatial memory. *Neuroscience.* 132(2): 261–71.

Smith A. C., et al. (2009). A Bayesian statistical analysis of behavioral facilitation associated with deep brain stimulation. *J Neurosci Meth.* 183: 267–76.

Smith R., Thayer J. F., et al. (2017). The hierarchical basis of neurovisceral integration. *Neurosci Biobehav Rev.* 75: 274–96.

Smyser C. D., et al. (2010). Longitudinal analysis of neural network development in preterm infants. *Cereb Cortex.* 20: 2852–62.

Snyder A. Z. (2016). Intrinsic brain activity and resting state networks. In: Pfaff D. W., Volkow N. D.) *Neuroscience in the 21st Century* (2nd edition, volume 3). New York, NY: Springer Verlag, pp. 1626–83.

Solovey G., et al. (2012). Self-regulated dynamical criticality in human ECoG. *Front Integr Neurosci.* 6:44

(2015). Loss of consciousness is associated with stabilization of cortical activity. *J Neurosci.* 35(30): 10866–77.

Spiteri T., et al. (2010). The role of the estrogen receptor alpha in the medial amygdala and ventromedial nucleus of the hypothalamus in social recognition, anxiety and aggression. *Behav Brain Res.* 210(2): 211–20.

Spiteri T., Ogawa S., Musatov S., Pfaff D. W., Agmo A. (2012). The role of the estrogen receptor α in the medial preoptic area in sexual incentive motivation, proceptivity and receptivity, anxiety, and wheel running in female rats. *Behav Brain Res.* 230(1): 11–20.

Sporns O., Tononi G., Edelman G. M. (2000) Connectivity and complexity: the relationship between neuroanatomy and brain dynamics. *Neural Netw.* 13(8–9):909–22.

Sporns O. (2011). *Networks of the Brain.* Cambridge: MIT Press.

Squire L. R., et al. (Eds.), *Fundamental Neuroscience.* San Diego, CA: Academic Press (Elsevier).

Stallings M. C., et al. (1996). Genetic and environmental structure of the Tridimensional Personality Questionnaire: three or four temperament dimensions? *J Pers Social Psychol.* 70(1): 127–40.

Stam C. J. (2014). Modern network science of neurological disorders. *Nat Rev Neurosci.* 15(10): 683–95.

Stanski D. R., Shafer S. (2005). Measuring depth of anesthesia. In: Miller R. D. (Ed.), *Miller's Anesthesia* (6th edition). Philadelphia, PA: Churchill-Livingstone, pp. 1227–64.

Starzl T. E., Taylor C. W., Magoun H. W. (1951). Ascending conduction in reticular activating system, with special reference to the diencephalon. *J Neurophysiol.* 14: 461–77.

Stauffer W. R., Lak A., Kobayashi S., Schultz W. (2016). Components and characteristics of the dopamine reward utility signal. *J Comp Neurol.* 524(8): 1699–711.

Steriade M., (2003). The corticothalamic system in sleep. *Front Biosci.* 8:d878–899.

Steriade M., Paré D., Bouhassira D., Deschênes M., Oakson G. (1989). Phasic activation of lateral geniculate and perigeniculate thalamic neurons during sleep with ponto-geniculo-occipital waves. *J Neurosci.* 9(7): 2215–29.

Steriade M., Datta S., Pare D., Oakson G., Curro Dossi R. C. (1990). Neuronal activation in brain-stem cholinergic nuclei related to tonic activation processes in thalamocortical systems. *J Neurosci.* 10: 2541–59.

Steriade M., Dossi R. C., Pare D., Oakson G. (1991). Fast oscillations (20–40 Hz) in thalamocortical systems and their potentiation by mesopontine cholinergic nuclei in the cat. *Proc Natl Acad Sci.* 88: 4396–400.

Steriade M., McCormick D. A., Sejnowski T. J. (1993). Thalamocortical oscillations in the sleeping and aroused brain. *Science.* 262: 679–85.

Stevens J. S. et al. (2017). Amygdala reactivity and anterior cingulated habituation predict posttraumatic stress disorder syndrome maintenance after acute civilian trauma. *Biol Psychiatry.* 81: 1023–9.

Studer L. (2012). Derivation of dopaminergic neurons from pluripotent stem cells. *Prog Brain Res.* 200: 243–63.

(2017). Strategies for bringing stem cell-derived dopamine neurons to the clinic-The NYSTEM trial. *Prog Brain Res.* 230: 191–212.

Sundermann E. E., Maki P. M., Bishop J. R. (2010). A review of estrogen receptor alpha gene (ESR1) polymorphisms, mood, and cognition. *Menopause.* 17(4): 874–86.

Suzuki D. T. (1960). *Introduction to Zen Buddhism.* London: Rider & Co.

Swanson L. W. (1982). The projections of the ventral tegmental area and adjacent regions: a combined fluorescent retrograde tracer and immunofluorescence study in the rat. *Brain Res Bull.* 9: 321–53.

Swanson L. W., Hartman B. K. (1974). The central adrenergic system. *J Comp Neurol.* 163: 467–506.

Tabansky I., Quinkert A. W., Rahman N., et al. (2014). Temporally-patterned deep brain stimulation in a mouse model of multiple traumatic brain injury. *Behav Brain Res.* 273:123–32.

Tabansky I., Stern J. N., Pfaff D. W. (2015). Implications of epigenetic variability within a cell population for "Cell Type" classification. *Front Behav Neurosci.* 9:342.

Tabansky I., et al. (2018). Molecular profiling of reticular gigantocellularis neurons indicates that eNOS modulates environmentally dependent levels of arousal. *Proc Natl Acad Sci.* 115: 6900–6909. doi: 10.1073/pnas.1806123115.

Taheri S., Zeitzer J. M., Mignot E. (2002). The role of hypocretins (orexins) in sleep regulation and narcolepsy. *Ann Rev Neurosci.* 25: 283–313.

Takahashi J. S. (2016). Molecular architecture of the circadian clock in mammals. In: Sassone-Corsi P., Christen Y., (Eds.), *A Time for Metabolism and Hormones [Internet].* Cham (CH): Springer.

Takamori S., Rhee J. S., Rosenmund C., Jahn R. (2001). Identification of differentiation-associated brain-specific phosphate transporter as a second vesicular glutamate transporter (VGLUT2). *J Neurosci.* 21:RC182.

Takigawa M., Mogenson G. J. (1977). A study of inputs to antidromically identified neurons of the locus coeruleus. *Brain Res.* 135: 217–30.

Tan K., Le Douarin N. M. (1991). Development of the nuclei and cell migration in the medulla oblongata. Application of the quail-chick chimera system. *Anat Embryol (Berl).* 183(4): 321–43.

Tang W., et al. (2017). Dynamic connectivity modulates local activity in the core regions of the default-mode network. *PNAS.* 114: 9713–18.

Taylor P. N., Wang Y., Kaiser M. (2017). Within brain area tractography suggests local modularity using high resolution connectomics. *Sci Rep.* 7:39859. doi: 10.1038/srep39859.

Thibaut A., et al. (2017). Controlled clinical trial of repeated prefrontal tDCS in patients with chronic minimally conscious state. *Brain Inj.* 31(4): 466–74.

Thompson R. H., Swanson L. W. (2003). Structural characterization of a hypothalamic visceromotor pattern generator network. *Brain Res Rev.* 41: 153–202.

Thor D. H., Wainwright K. L., Holloway W. R. (1982). Persistence of attention to a novel conspecific: some developmental variables in laboratory rats. *Dev Psychobiol.* 15(1): 1–8.

Tong L. (2005). Acetyl-coenzyme A carboxylase: crucial metabolic enzyme and attractive target for drug discovery. *Cell Mol Life Sci.* 62:1784–803.

Tonge D. A., de Burgh H. T., Docherty R., et al. (2012). Fibronectin supports neurite outgrowth and axonal regeneration of adult brain neurons in vitro. *Brain Res.* 1453:8–16.

Tononi G., Edelman G. M. (1998) Consciousness and complexity. *Science.* 282(5395): 1846–51.

Top D., Young M. W. (2017). Coordination between differentially regulated circadian clocks generates rhythmic behavior. *Cold Spring Harb Perspect Biol.* pii:a033589. doi: 10.1101/cshperspect.a033589.

Trofimova I., Robbins T. W. (2016). Temperament and arousal systems: a new synthesis of differential psychology and functional neurochemistry. *Neurosci Biobehav Rev.* 64: 382–402.

Tsunematsu T., Kilduff T. S., Boyden E. S. et al. (2011) Article II. Acute optogenetic silencing of orexin/hypocretin neurons induces slow-wave sleep in mice. *J Neurosci.* 31(29): 10529–39. doi: 10.1523/JNEUROSCI.0784-11.2011.

Turney S. G., Bridgman P. C. (2005). Laminin stimulates and guides axonal outgrowth via growth cone myosin II activity. *Nat Neurosci.* 8:717–19.

Valentino R. J., Foote S. L. (1988). Corticotropin-releasing hormone increases tonic but not sensory-evoked activity of noradrenergic locus coeruleus neurons in unanesthetized rats. *J Neurosci.* 8(3): 1016–25.

Valentino R. J., Foote S. L., Aston-Jones G. (1983). Corticotropin-releasing factor activates noradrenergic neurons of the locus coeruleus. *Brain Res.* 270(2): 363–7.

Valentino R. J., Page M., Van Bockstaele E., Aston-Jones G. (1992). Corticotropin-releasing factor innervation of the locus coeruleus region: distribution of fibers and sources of input. *Neuroscience.* 48: 689–705.

Valentino R. J., Rudoy C., Saunders A., Liu X. B., Van Bockstaele E. J. (2001). Corticotropin-releasing factor is preferentially colocalized with excitatory rather than inhibitory amino acids in axon terminals in the peri-locus coeruleus region. *Neuroscience.* 106(2): 375–84.

Valverde F. (1961). Reticular formation of the pons and medulla oblongata; a Golgi study. *J Comp Neurol.* 116: 71–99.

(1962). Reticular formation of the albino rat's brain stem. *J Comp Neurol.* 119: 25–49.

van Someren E., Cluydts R. (2017). Sleep regulation and insomnia. In Pfaff D. W., Volkow N. D., *Neuroscience in the 21st Century* (2nd edition, volume 3). Heidelberg, New York: Springer, pp. 2289–316.

van Swinderen B., Greenspan R. J. (2003). Salience modulates 20–30 Hz brain activity in Drosophila. *Nat Neurosci.* 6(6): 579–86.

Vanderwolf C. H., Stewart D. J. (1998). Thalamic control of neocortical activation: a critical re-evaluation. *Brain Res Bull.* 20: 529–38.

Vasquez-Vivar J., Kalyanaraman B., Martasek P., et al. (1998). Superoxide generation by endothelial nitric oxide synthase: the influence of cofactors. *Proc Natl Acad Sci U S A.* 95:9220–5.

Vazey E. M., Aston-Jones G. (2014). Designer receptor manipulations reveal a role of the locus coeruleus noradrenergic system in isoflurane general anesthesia. *Proc Natl Acad Sci U S A.* 111(10): 3859–64.

Vertes R. P., Martin G. F., Waltzer R. (1986). An autoradiographic analysis of ascending projections from the medullary reticular formation in the rat. *Neuroscience.* 19:873–98.

Villablanca J., Salinas-Zeballos M. E. (1972). Sleep-wakefulness, EEG and behavioral studies of chronic cats without the thalamus: the 'athalamic' cat. *Arch Ital Biol.* 110: 383–411.

Villano I., Messina A., Valenzano A. et al. (2017). Basal forebrain cholinergic system and orexin neurons: effects on attention. *Front Behav Neurosci.* 11:10. doi: 10.3389/fnbeh.2017.00010.

Vincent J. L., et al. (2007). Intrinsic functional architecture in the anesthetized monkey brain. *Nature.* 447: 46–7.

Von Economo J. (1926). *Handbuch der Normalen und Pathologischen Physiologie.* Berlin: Springer, pp. 591–610.

Vosshall L. B, et al. (1994). Block in nuclear localization of period protein by a second clock mutation, timeless. *Science*. 263(5153): 1606–9.

Vosshall L. B., Young M. W. (1995). Circadian rhythms in Drosophila can be driven by period expression in a restricted group of central brain cells. *Neuron*. 15(2): 345–60.

Vujovic N., et al. (2015). Projections from the subparaventricular zone define four channels of output from the circadian timing system. *J Comp Neurol*. 523(18): 2714–37.

Waid D. K., Chell M., El-Fakahany E. E. (2000). M(2) and M(4) muscarinic receptor subtypes couple to activation of endothelial nitric oxide synthase. *Pharmacology*. 61:37–42.

Wang C., et al. (1996). Testosterone replacement therapy improves mood in hypogonadal men – a clinical research center study. *J Clin Endocrinol Metab*. 81(10): 3578–83.

Wang S., et al. (2017). The human amygdala parametrically encodes the intensity of specific facial emotions and their categorical ambiguity. *Nat Commun*. 21(8): 14821. doi: 10.1038/ncomms14821.

Wannez S., et al. (2017). Prevalence of coma-recovery scale-revised signs of consciousness in patients in minimally conscious state. *Neuropsychol Rehabil*. 11: 1–10.

Watson C. J., Lydic R., Baghdoyan H. A. (2011). Sleep duration varies as a function of glutamate and GABA in rat pontine reticular formation. *J Neurochem*. 118(4): 571–80.

Weber F., Yan Y. (2016). Circuit-based interrogation of sleep control. *Nature*. 538: 51–61.

Webster H. H., Jones B. E. (1988). Neurotoxic lesions of the dorsolateral pontomesencephalic tegmentum-cholinergic cell area in the cat. II. Effects upon sleep-waking states. *Brain Res*. 458(2): 285–302.

Weil Z. M., et al. (2010). Impact of generalized brain arousal on sexual behavior. *Proc Natl Acad Sci*. 107(5): 2265–70.

Weinberger J. (2018). *A Brief History of Unconscious Processes*. New Haven, CT: Guilford Press

Weitzman E. D. (1981). Sleep and its disorders. *Annu Rev Neurosci*. 4: 381–417.

Wenk G. L., Stoehr J. D., Quintana G., Mobley S., Wiley R. G. (1994). Behavioral, biochemical, histological, and electrophysiological effects of 192 IgG-saporin injections into the basal forebrain of rats. *J Neurosci*. 14: 5986–95.

Williams K. M., Mong J. A. (2017). Methamphetamine and ovarian steroid responsive cells in the posteriodorsal medial amygdala are required for methamphetamine-enhanced proceptive behaviors. *Science Rep*. 2017 7:39817.

Winsky-Sommerer R., Yamanaka A., Diano S., et al., (2004). Interaction between the corticotrophin-releasing factor system and hypocretins (orexins): a novel circuit mediating stress response. *J Neurosci*. 24: 11439–48.

Wood S. K., Valentino R. J. (2017). The brain norepinephrine system, stress and cardiovascular vulnerability. *Neurosci Biobehav Rev*. 74(Pt B):393–400.

Wu H. B., Stavarache M., Pfaff D. W., Kow L. M. (2007). Arousal of cerebral cortex electroencephalogram consequent to high-frequency stimulation of ventral medullary reticular formation. *Proc Natl Acad Sci U S A*. 104(46): 18292–6.

Wu H., Stavarache M., Pfaff D. W., Kow L. (2007). Arousal of cerebral cortex electroencephalogram consequent to high-frequency stimulation of ventral medullary reticular formation. *Proc Natl Acad Sci*. 104(46): 18292–6.

Xia Y., Tsai A. L., Berka V., Zweier J. L. (1998). Superoxide generation from endothelial nitric-oxide synthase. A Ca2+/calmodulin-dependent and tetrahydrobiopterin regulatory process. *J Biol Chem*. 273:25804–8.

Xu C., Datta S., Wu M., Alreja M. (2004). Hippocampal theta rhythm is reduced by suppression of the H-current in septohippocampal GABAergic neurons. *Eur J Neurosci*. 19: 2299–309.

Yackle K., et al. (2017). Breathing control center neurons that promote arousal in mice. *Science*. 355: 1411–15.

Yamanaka A. et al. (2003). Hypothalamic orexin neurons regulate arousal according to energy balance in mice. *Neuron*. 38(5): 701–13.

Yanofsky N. (2016). Paradoxes, contradictions and the limits of science. *Sci Am.* 104: 166–78.

Yokota S., Oka T., Tsumori T., Nakamura S., Yasui Y. (2007). Glutamatergic neurons in the Kolliker-Fuse nucleus project to the rostral ventral respiratory group and phrenic nucleus. A combined retrograde tracing and in situ hybridization study in the rat. *Neurosci Res.* 59: 342–6.

Yokota S., et al. (2015). Respiratory-related outputs of glutamatergic, hypercapnia-responsive parabrachial neurons in mice. *J Comp Neurol.* 523(6): 907–20.

Yoshida Y., et al. (2001). Fluctuation of extracellular hypocretin-1 (orexin A) levels in the rat in relation to the light-dark cycle and sleep-wake activities. *Eur J Neurosci.* 14(7): 1075–81.

Young J. W. (2009). Dopamine D1 and D2 receptor family contributions to modafinil-induced wakefulness. *J Neurosci.* 29: 2663–5.

Young M. W. (2002). Big ben rings in a lesson on biological clocks. *Neuron.* 36: 1001–5.

Young M. W., Kay S. A. (2001). Time zones: a comparative genetics of circadian clocks. *Nat Rev Genet.* 2: 702–15.

Zaborszky L., Cullinan W. E. (1989). Hypothalamic axons terminate on forebrain cholinergic neurons: an ultrastructural double-labeling study using PHA-L tracing and ChAT immunocytochemistry. *Brain Res.* 479: 177–84.

Zaborszky L., et al. (2005). Three-dimensional chemoarchitecture of the basal forebrain: Spatially specific association of cholinergic and calcium binding protein-containing neurons. *Neuroscience.* 136: 697–713.

Zaborszky L., Pol A. V. D., Gyengesi E., (2012). The basal forebrain cholinergic projection system in mice. In: Watson C., Paxinos G., Puelles L. (Eds.), *The Mouse Nervous System* (1st edition). Amsterdam: Elsevier, pp. 684–718.

Zaborszky L., et al. (2015). Neurons in the basal forebrain project to the cortex in a complex topographic organization that reflects corticocortical connectivity patterns: an experimental study based on retrograde tracing and 3D reconstruction. *Cerebr Cortex.* 25: 118–37.

Zagha E., McCormick D. A. (2014). Neural control of brain state. *Curr Opin Neurobiol.* 29: 178–86.

Zavalko I. et al. (2012). Hypersomnia due to bilateral thalamic lesions: unexpected response to Modafinil. *Eur J Neurol.* 19: 125–37.

Zeitzer J. M., Nishino S., Mignot E. (2006). The neurobiology of hypocretins (orexins), narcolepsy and related therapeutic interventions. *Trends Pharmacol Sci.* 27(7): 368–74.

Zeman A. (2001). Consciousness *Brain.* 124: 1263–89.

(2002). *Consciousness, a User's Guide.* New Haven, CT: Yale University Press.

Zemlan F. P., Kow L. M., Pfaff D. W. (1983). Effect of interruption of bulbospinal pathways on lordosis, posture, and locomotion. *Exp Neurol.* 81(1): 177–94.

Zemlan F. P., Behbehani M. M., Beckstead R. M. (1984). Ascending and descending projections from nucleus reticularis magnocellularis and nucleus reticularis gigantocellularis: an autoradiographic and horseradish peroxidase study in the rat. *Brain Res.* 292:207–20.

Zhao W., Becker J. B. (2010). Sensitization enhances acquisition of cocaine self-administration in female rats: estradiol further enhances cocaine intake after acquisition. *Horm Behav.* 58(1): 8–12.

Zhao X., et al. (2014). Nuclear receptors rock around the clock. *EMBO Rep.* 15(5): 518–28.

Zhou J., et al. (2009). Arousal-related reticular neurons during reduced oxygen tension: resilience and recovery of electrical activity. *Dev Neurosci.* 31(4): 255–8.

Zoubina E. V., Smith P. G. (2003). Expression of estrogen receptors alpha and beta by sympathetic ganglion neurons projecting to the proximal urethra of female rats. *J Urol.* 169: 382–5.

Index

accumbens nucleus, 53
acetylcholine, 16, 26, 57, 66, 67, 72, 84
ACh, 67
action potentials, 29, 31, 35, 68, 69, 72, 73, 81, 119
activation of neurons, 8
Adam Zeman, 112
ADHD, 25, 122
adrenal glands, 19, 89
adrenaline, 50
adrenergic neurons, 17
Adrian Owen, 104
adults, 25
agent consciousness, 110
aggression, 4, 19, 21, 58, 80, 81, 82, 83, 84, 85, 86, 91, 120
aggressive behavior, 19, 20, 80, 81, 82, 83, 84, 86, 91, 93
aging, 25, 122
Albert-Lazlo Barabasi, 116
alcohol, 25
alertness, 20, 80, 82, 84, 85, 86
Alex Proekt, 23, 34, 96, 116
α-ERKO, 17
Alzheimer's, 4, 25, 122
amino acids, 8, 42, 50, 51, 55, 58, 59, 60
Amos Maritan, 23
Amos Tversky, 94
amphibia, 35
Amy Wells Quinkert, 73, 105
amygdala, 25, 40, 43, 44, 46, 52, 53, 55, 69, 80, 86, 87, 88, 89, 90, 91, 92
amygdala neurons, 89, 90
amygdaloid neurons, 89
Ana Ribeiro, 100
ancient forebrain, 29, 39, 44, 52
Andrew Hudson, 96
androgen receptor, 85
anesthesia, 1, 3, 4, 11, 12, 13, 21, 25, 30, 31, 59, 72, 73, 75, 94, 95, 96, 97, 98, 106, 108, 113, 119, 121
anesthetics, 12, 94, 95, 96, 98

anesthetization, 11, 98
anger, 6, 21, 83, 85
animals, 1, 3, 4, 5, 6, 7, 9, 11, 13, 14, 18, 19, 22, 23, 26, 27, 28, 29, 31, 33, 40, 41, 46, 49, 54, 57, 58, 60, 61, 63, 64, 65, 74, 77, 81, 82, 83, 84, 85, 87, 88, 89, 90, 91, 92, 93, 100, 104, 105, 110, 111, 112, 115, 119, 120, 121
Ansgar Beckermann, 109
antibodies, 39
antidepressants, 44
anti-histamines, 58
anxiety, 17, 19, 86, 88, 90, 91
anxiolytics, 82
A/P systems of communication, 1, 2, 3, 5, 6, 8, 9, 10, 27, 32, 36, 38, 46, 48, 49, 68, 70, 71, 79, 90, 106, 115, 116, 118, 121, 122
apes, 111
AR, 63, 85
Aristotle, 48
arousal, 1, 2, 3, 4, 5, 6, 7, 8, 9, 10, 11, 12, 13, 14, 15, 16, 17, 18, 19, 20, 21, 23, 24, 25, 26, 27, 28, 30, 31, 32, 33, 34, 35, 36, 37, 38, 39, 40, 41, 43, 44, 45, 46, 47, 48, 49, 51, 52, 53, 54, 55, 56, 57, 58, 59, 61, 62, 63, 64, 65, 66, 67, 69, 70, 71, 72, 73, 74, 75, 79, 81, 82, 83, 84, 86, 90, 91, 92, 93, 95, 100, 101, 102, 103, 104, 105, 112, 113, 115, 116, 117, 119, 120, 122
arousal assay, 11, 18
arousal mechanisms, 3, 22, 25, 41, 48, 115
arousal systems, 1, 3, 7, 8, 9, 10, 11, 21, 27, 46, 67, 69, 71, 79, 86, 117, 120, 122
Arthur Loewy, 8
atrophy, 69

attack, 19, 80, 81, 82, 121
attention-dependent behavioral circuits, 40
auditory aspects, 12, 18, 20, 22, 32, 69, 75, 77, 86, 87, 90, 102, 103, 112
auditory system, 22
autism spectrum disorders, 25
autonomic arousal, 92
autonomic functions, 43, 46, 112
autonomic nerves, 43
autonomic nervous system, 15, 35, 83, 84, 88
autonomic regulation, 41
autonomic signals, 49
autonomic sympathetic activity, 12
autonomic system, 32, 83, 84
autoradiography, 50, 51
autoreceptors, 56
awakening, 41, 102
awareness, 3, 8, 33, 68, 69, 71, 75, 76, 94, 96, 102, 103, 104, 108, 110, 112, 113, 114
axons, 1, 4, 5, 8, 9, 11, 16, 17, 28, 30, 32, 33, 34, 35, 37, 41, 42, 44, 46, 49, 51, 53, 55, 56, 57, 59, 60, 66, 67, 70, 71, 72, 78, 87, 88, 116, 119, 121, 122

balance, 10, 16, 60
Barabási-Albert scale-free model, 121
Barbara Jones, 21, 51, 67
Barbiturates, 94
Barry Peterson, 33
basal forebrain, 4, 9, 17, 27, 33, 36, 49, 50, 51, 52, 53, 57, 58, 66, 67, 70, 72, 79, 84, 105, 116, 117, 119
basal ganglia, 69, 71, 76, 104, 105
bauplan, 35
BDNF, 67